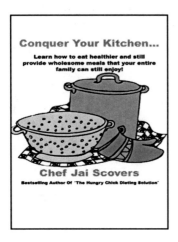

On Sale Now...

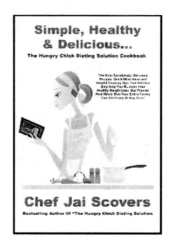

"Simple, Healthy& Delicious..."

The Hungry Chick Dieting Solution Cookbook!

Chef Jai Scovers shares her favorite most satisfying, delicious recipes, quick meal ideas and helpful cooking tips in her full color, new cookbook... "Simple, Healthy & Delicious"

That will not only help you maintain your healthy weight loss, but provide real meals that your entire family can still enjoy at any time!

Buy Your Copy Right Now!

You Are Not Alone…

About two and a half years ago, I got something shocking in the mail. As I opened the envelope, I almost screamed. There I was, standing at my front door, going through the mail, and suddenly, I found myself staring at the photo of something that left me absolutely speechless. I actually stood there at my front door with my mouth hung open in sheer terror.

For a moment, I panicked! Looking around to see if anyone had seen me and my reactions, I quickly closed the front door and reached for my telephone. As I dialed a very familiar number, I could hardly breathe as I listened to the phone ring. Finally, she answered. Good.

As I said "hello," she knew in an instant that it was me and she had even been expecting my call. I took a deep breath and I asked her the one question that we all have probably asked someone, at some point in our lives, "When did you take that picture?" It was the same picture that I was still holding in my hand from the mail.

She laughed and said, "At your cousin's birthday party." The truth is that I wasn't doing anything really special in the picture. I was just standing around talking. But, I was horrified by the way that the picture made me look. As I stared at the picture, the only thing that I kept thinking was that, "I really do need to lose some weight."

My friend didn't mean any harm. I knew that. Yet, for me, I still felt like the world was ending all around me. It didn't help that when I thanked her, she said that she was glad that she had sent it. She then said, "You looked so cute." I didn't think so. I was literally crushed.

1

We have all have been there. It's that dreadful moment when someone takes a picture of you, and in this day and age, posted it to the internet, or on Facebook, without showing you or telling you about it first. When you finally do see it, you just want to cry. That's because candid pictures will tell the real story about how we really look every day. That's why we hate them.

It's not that you look bad, it's just that, well, you just do not look good either. The worst part is trying to figure out how to ask your friend, or your family member, to get rid of that picture without sounding harsh or angry? There simply isn't an easy way to do it. There isn't.

At that point, you will start to remember how you have a closet full of clothes, but never have anything to wear that fits right. How many times have you stood in the back whenever someone asked a group of you to take a picture? What happens when you can't hide?

How many times do you have to adjust your clothes just to stand up or move around a room? It becomes almost a reflex, like trying to catch yourself when you are about to fall. Worst of all, you have to do it. If you didn't, you would feel very self-conscious. I know that I used to, before I lost 18 pounds and managed to keep it off.

How many times have you seen someone thinner than you and you start to think to yourself that she can probably eat whatever she wants? Luck chick. She never seems to gain a pound. Why not you? It is not fair.

In college, you might have been so thin. You could eat almost anything and never gain a single pound. Now, you can't even walk past the bakery section in the supermarket without gaining five pounds from just the smell of the cupcakes. That's really not fair!

As I hung up the phone with my friend, I looked at the picture again. I felt horrible. At that moment, right then and there, I decided that I was going to lose weight. I was going to change the way that I was eating and focus on getting fit again. I had to do this for me.

Within weeks, I went to see my doctor and I was told that I could stand to lose a few pounds. The question, at hand, was how? Sure, she gave me a few tips to lose some weight, but, I needed to learn how to keep that weight off once I lost it. At that point, I had already tried almost every weight loss plan and program on the market and I still hadn't found one that was right for me.

Most weight loss plans, I have found, tend to talk down to you, like you don't know anything. With some plans, they make a whole bunch of empty promises. With other plans, they require you to make some very expensive changes to your life and some just don't work at all.

According to a recent survey of women, at any given time, over 50 percent of all women are on a diet. If that is the case, why are so many of these women still overweight? I didn't want to be on my own, but, I wasn't willing to risk my life or long term health on a fad diet, which only works for a little while, to do it. So, I kept looking. I wanted a plan that wouldn't force me to give up everything that, as a chef, I love about food.

The next week at the supermarket, in my determination not to give up, I bought a whole bunch of healthy snacks.

I started drinking diet sodas. A friend told me to go the book store and pick up this one book that promised me that I'd be skinny. Promises. Promises.

Within a week, I realized that I was making one of the biggest mistakes of my life. I was starving, so I quit. It simply wasn't working. Instead of being a skinny chick, I was a hungry one. I was starving. I needed to do something else and I needed to do it quickly. I had to.

As you know, the hunger games, when you are trying to lose weight, become very real and every last snack becomes a losing battle. I was so afraid of gaining any more weight and I was even more afraid that I wouldn't be able to lose any of the weight that I already had.

I knew in my heart that there were other women, like you, out there who were just like me. The question, then, is what do we do about it? It isn't like you and I aren't trying to lose the weight. We just don't know how. Nobody ever told us how to lose weight, and more importantly, how to keep it off for good. I began to wonder did any of these diet plans even know how to.

Still, my determination remained strong. So I kept looking for something that works. What I soon learned was that any weight loss plan that expects you to change everything about your life within a few weeks is guaranteed to fail. The ones that I tried already have.

As a result, I found myself hungrier than ever and I was miserable. I wanted to eat like I used to, because with this dieting thing, nothing seemed to satisfy my appetite. When you are hungry, you eat, but what you eat is not always what and how you are supposed to eat. Trust me, we all have been there. There you are hungrier than ever, but still desperately trying to lose weight.

At this point, you might have already tried the pills, the cream, and even, learned to like cabbage soup. You have skipped breakfast, sometimes lunch and skimped on dinner. You have already tried drinking lots of water and eating carrots and learned to like celery. You will do just about anything just to see a size six again.

You have never met anyone named Atkins, but you tried the diet. That's just like you have never been to South Beach, so you don't even know if that diet book is really from there. Still, you tried it anyway.

The plan that you saw on Good Morning America, you tried it. The plan that your sister's best friend swears by, you have tried that too. You now hate her because you don't know how she managed to lose so much weight!

The box, that your meal plans came in, probably tastes better than the actual meal. Your before and after pictures still look like the same picture with a different outfit. You tried running, but, in the end, it was only for the ice cream truck. Dinner is often your hardest meal, because you are often too tired to cook and will eat just about anything that is easy or convenient.

With most diet plans and weight loss programs, I use the words interchangeably; I learned that I couldn't just change what I was eating. I had to change my life around to meet the weight loss program's extraordinary needs. I did this even when the only thing that I needed was a weight loss program that would meet my needs. That's why I wasn't losing weight.

I soon began to realize that losing weight isn't the same as joining a twelve step program, where the first thing that you have to do is to admit that you have a problem, and suddenly, you are on the road to recovery. You already know that you want to lose weight. The question is how to do it safely and effectively? Then, keep it off!

Sure, during the winter months, you can hide behind a bulky sweater that your grandmother gave you, but in the summer, the truth comes out and you feel embarrassed by it. That is until the next weight loss plan, pill or gimmick comes along and you start the cycle of yo-yo dieting all over again. Yes, I said yo-yo dieting.

Yo-yo dieting is a complicated way of losing weight. That's where when you are trying to lose weight, you successfully lose some weight, and then, you gain it all back, all over again. Then, you manage to lose this weight all over again on your next diet. But, like a yo-yo, the weight comes right back. This is very frustrating and can lead to poor eating habits for many women. It can also be damaging to your good health.

At that point you, you can try again or you can give up and give in to those extra unhealthy and unwanted pounds. At least that's what the world expects us to do. Society tells us that we are losing the war on obesity and when you are any size above a two. You simply aren't good enough. You can't even control your weight.

That's the point where you learn to do math. The two piece bikini becomes a one piece swim suit in the summer. You, then, add a top to it and some shorts or a wraparound. What started out as two piece swim suit has multiplied into a full outfit. In the summer, it really is too hot for all of that extra clothing, but you are too embarrassed to wear anything less than that.

Having worked everywhere from the world famous Showboat Casino and Hotel in Atlantic City, New Jersey to the famed Stephen Starr restaurants, you should know that I enjoy a good meal just like you do. I used to live to eat, but I still love to cook. It always has been this way and always will be. But, even as a chef, what I have learned is that food doesn't have to control my life and it shouldn't be allowed to control yours.

You shouldn't have to spend countless hours worrying about what will happen if you eat this and what will happen if you eat that. Eventually, you will not eat anything at all, you will be too afraid that you'll gain weight and be fat. Whoever said that you should have to starve yourself just to lose a few extra pounds?

The truth is that we all want to look better, feel better, eat better and have much more energy. But, why should you have to give up all of your favorite foods to do it? Why should you have to deny yourself the very things that make you happy to achieve this? The truth is you shouldn't have to give up everything that you love.

I was at this point when I stumbled across the solution to my dieting problems and yours. It helped me to lose my 18 pounds. I learned that it wasn't just the diet plans that are the problems. It is you and I. We have found ourselves believing in these weight loss plans, more than we have ever believed in ourselves.

We fed into the belief that without them, we wouldn't be happy. In the end, we stopped doing the one thing that allowed us to get this far, we stopped loving who we are! We stopped loving what made us special.

By allowing a weight loss program to determine our sense of self-worth, we lost the motivation to do what will make us happy. We lost the motivation to take care of ourselves. Eating healthier doesn't mean eating less, it means making more nutritional choices in the foods that we already know and love.

Even if you never wear even a size six again, you should still be happy. Even if you never own a pair of skinny jeans, you should still feel good about yourself. This constant war with our bodies had only made it easier to constantly eat things that aren't good for us. We stopped being good to us and we stopped eating the very foods that are good for us.

By falling back in love with me, I gained the motivation and confidence to finally lose my 18 pounds and keep them off. Not just for a few months, but for two years now. How? I learned how to eat when I am hungry and I only eat when I should and I never overdo it. Sounds simple? That's because it is and I will show you how.

Trust me, as a woman, I understand what is like to want to lose that extra weight and you feel like you can't or you just don't know how. I understand that inside of every woman, including you, you feel like there is a healthier, slimmer version trying to get out. You just didn't know how to make this happen. I can help you.

The problem is, the woman that I want to show you, using this solution, might not be a size two. She might be a healthy size eight. By changing how you look at food, using simple things to balance your diet and adding a few simple "exercises" to your day, you can finally reach your ideal or goal weight and become the person that you have always wanted to be.

I just don't want you to waste another minute of your life trying to live with that extra weight, and then, having to make excuses for it. Also, maybe, I should warn you that this book isn't going to be some college dissertation on the merits of weight loss. There is no scientific mumbo jumbo that is meant to confuse you.

My goal is to be as inspiring, educational and informative as possible. I want this to be a real woman to woman conversation on what truly works in becoming healthier. This is a step-by-step guide for women, like you, who have tried to lose weight on other diet plans and weight loss programs, to finally lose that weight, and then, show you how to keep it off for good.

You should also know that this will be the only diet book that I will ever write. The number one way that you can always tell that some diets really don't work is because every couple of years, they are always coming out with a "new" one. Why wasn't the first one good enough?

They already know that the average person tries up to four "new" diets a year, so by designing their diet to fail, or only work for a little bit, they can make more money offering you a new and "improved" one. Not this one!

Also, I tried to keep the chapters and the paragraphs shorter and easier to read. This isn't supposed to be a lecture or your high school history book! If you wanted a case study, I am afraid that you have come to the wrong place. I am here to help you, not bore you to death. We all make mistakes. I might have made one or two. Nobody is perfect. Forgive me as you will learn to forgive yourself for struggling with your weight all of these years.

What I want to share with you will give you the first chance to stop struggling with your weight and the first chance that you have ever had to start living again. We can't afford to lose the fight on obesity. That's why I want to show you how to win the war to be healthier. You owe that much to yourself and to your family.

As a trained gourmet chef and a graduate of the world renown Restaurant School at Walnut Hill College, healthy eating is not just something that I know; it has become a big part of my life. Make it a part of yours.

So take a moment to congratulate yourself. What I am about to show you is the most proven, safe and effective way to help you achieve your ideal or goal weight. At this very moment, right now, you are now only a few weeks away from a healthier, slimmer you.

Now that you have taken the challenge to change your life, I guarantee you that the results will be absolutely remarkable. It's something you will be very proud of. I really do want this to be the very last diet or weight loss book that you will ever buy for yourself.

Allow The Hungry Chick Dieting Solution to change your life the same way that it did for me. You should know that you are now a hungry chick and hungry chicks should never go hungry…

The Hungry Chick Dieting Solution

Whoever Said That You Should Have To Starve Yourself Just To Lose A Few Unwanted Pounds?

Chef Jai Scovers

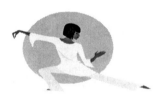

J. Scovers Healthy Solutions

Disclaimer: Losing weight depends on your commitment to eating healthier and exercising. Your results will differ based on your weight loss efforts.

That's why you should ALWAYS consult YOUR primary care doctor before starting any weight loss, weight management, fitness or health related program, even if it's written or has been organized by a professional or expert in that field. No one but your primary care doctor knows your medical history.

Your health is your most important asset. Please don't risk it by ignoring or not seeking advice from your medical professional before starting anything that may put your health at risk. Results with any weight loss plan will vary. The information provided is a based on the author's beliefs and research.

The author and publisher specifically disclaims all responsibility for any liability, loss or risk, personal and otherwise, which is incurred as a direct or indirect consequence from the use or the application of any and/or all content from this book. This information is presented solely for its educational value only.

Table of Contents

Please Take A Moment To Read This...

This book is dedicated to God, who is the one that make everything possible. Of whom God gives much, much is required. Because, who we are is a gift from God and who we become is our gift to God.

I dedicate this book to my mother, Elizabeth Louise Clark, who is my daily inspiration to be a better person and to always do what I can to help other people live better and become better people for themselves.

I also dedicate this book to strong women everywhere. I don't care if you are a size zero or a fourteen. I understand your struggle to love yourself in a world, where because of our size, we often forget to love ourselves. You are beautiful in every single way.

Remember that as a real woman, you should always take the stones that have been thrown at you for not being thin enough, strong enough, pretty enough, smart enough, or even, talented enough and build a solid future for yourself with them.

Never let your struggles become your identity. Your struggles are a reminder of what you are capable of...

Chef Jai

The Dirty Little Secrets That Most Weight Loss Programs Never Want You To Ever Find Out...

When you wake up in the morning, has looking in the bathroom mirror become harder on your ever critical eyes? Maybe that's because you are not always seeing everything that is being reflected back at you.

Your efforts to lose weight are often rooted in your past and the way that you used to see yourself. It is also destroying every chance that you have ever truly had to lose those extra ten, twenty, or even, fifty pounds.

Rather through your ever critical eyes, your body has become a continuous collage of past and present experiences, based on forgotten praises or insults about your weight, constant worrying about being "fat" and your negative thoughts about never truly fitting in.

As a result, you will always come back to the same conclusion, "I do need to lose some weight." When it doesn't happen, you fall into a cycle of self-hatred because of something that is only partially your fault. Contrary to popular belief, you are only responsible for what you eat, not how your body reacts to it.

Still, in this weight conscious world, since early childhood and on, we have all developed a negative attitude towards being overweight. For most people, unless you look just like the model on the cover of a magazine, you really should try to lose some weight. Why not? The social rewards will be absolutely endless when it comes to being "skinny." You already know this, and more importantly, you deserve it. Right?

Just think about having a whole new wardrobe. The complements and the attention that you will receive will be endless. You not only want to look good, but you want to feel good too. You should know that the first casualty of your being overweight is your self-esteem.

The bigger that you are, the lower that your self-esteem is. This is something that many diet plans and programs have come to count on. If they didn't count on this, they would be out of business tomorrow.

To lose what ten, twenty, what the heck, fifty pounds, could do you some good right? Being big isn't necessary beautiful right? You can't continue to live your life longing for the days when abundant flesh becomes attractive again, can you?

It doesn't help that every day some new celebrity diet pretends to tell us how (you fill in the blank) lost all of her weight. You and I both could too if we had someone else preparing our meals and telling us what to do.

Instead, you ran out and joined the millions of Americans who have made dieting a "normal" way of life. You were drawn to the plans that make overconfident promises of a "thin, new you." Melt the fat away! Drop two dress sizes in one week! Burn off that belly fat!

Suddenly, you are on your way to becoming everything that you have ever dreamed of. All of this just to lose ten pounds. For all of the hassle, it might as well have been 100 pounds that you were trying to lose. The worst part is that your diet plan is counting on this. If you aren't struggling with your weight, you won't need their diet.

Many of these plans will never even tell you the truth about the hidden dangers found in this kind of dieting. They will never warn you about the health issues that many of these plans themselves can impose on your life. That's right; your plan could be hurting you.

Increasing evidence is showing that many of the health problems that these diet plans suggest can happen by being overweight, like headaches and muscle aches, are coming from the very diets themselves. If your plan relies on low calories, or have unusual ways to lose weight, you are already setting yourself up for failure.

Health officials are discovering that with the increasing pressure from the ever-growing number of diet plans coming on to the market, the people behind these plans and programs are more concerned with making a quick buck than helping you to effectively lose the weight that you truly need to lose, and then, to keep it off.

Many of these plans will promise you everything in their ads from rapid weight loss to claiming that a bulking agent, or a diet pill, will miraculously suppress your appetite when used in your diet. Some will say that you will be able to lose fat without having to limit the amount of calories in your diet. Where? I laugh at the ones that dare to say that you can lose weight without exercising.

Some plans require you to depend on their special prepackaged meals to lose weight, when they should be teaching you how to make better choices from the foods that you already eat now. The last thing that you will ever want to do is to sign an expensive contract for some long term plan that you won't need after this book.

You should never allow any diet to try and pass off salespersons as "qualified counselors" to give advice on nutrition and good health, while you are on their plan. This is dangerous since these "counselors" don't know your medical history and they are often being paid to push the plan and not really help you lose any weight, and then, teach you how to effectively keep it off. These misrepresentations could end up costing you dearly.

With over one billion people on this planet, who are overweight and 300 million of them obese, you should know that being overweight, specifically refers to an excessive amount weight that may come from muscles, bone, adipose (fat) tissue and water. When a person is obese, they are usually carrying an excessive amount of adipose tissue. Either way, both conditions will leave you at risk for type-2 diabetes, heart disease and cardiovascular problems, a stroke and some cancers.

When was the last time that a diet plan or weight loss program even explained the difference between being overweight and being obese to you, like I just did? Upset yet? You should be, but, wait, that's just the beginning of what I have to tell you.

I think that it is about time that I also tell you the other reasons why, and even, how every diet that you have ever been on, until now, has been designed to fail. That's because using some of these fad diets for even a day is like playing a deadly game of Russian roulette…

Here Are The Other Reasons Why Your Last Couple Of Diets Actually Failed...

The last time I quit a diet, it was because I was watching television late one night and I saw a program that came on about weight loss. In the infomercial, if you will, the woman was holding a piece of chocolate cake and she sprinkled what I call "fairy dust" on the cake and she said that's it. That was the key to losing more weight.

This was big news to me. My weight <u>loss</u> battle was suddenly over. Hallelujah! I immediately got up, went to the kitchen and sprinkled some powder sugar on a piece of cake and ate it. I think I gained five pounds that week from just trying that trick. It didn't work for me in any of the five times that I tried it and I am sure it wouldn't work for you either. Like your last diet, it will fail.

With every diet that I have ever been on, I always ended up feeling hungry. Working with food, I am always tempted to nibble, but, instead, on my last diet, I was starving. I soon learned that there are no magic tricks or short cuts to losing those extra, unhealthy and unwanted pounds. None. If there were, I would have found them a long time ago. I have been looking. That woman lied to me and she probably lied to you too.

The problem is that for you, the greatest lie that some of these plans probably have ever told you is that you can eat whatever you want and never gain weight. At one point, you probably told yourself this lie too.

The truth is that you weren't really able to eat anything that you wanted at any time in your life. You only thought that you could do that and here is the bottom line--you still can't and you never will be able to.

The truth is that your body is always changing. As you grow older, you will have to become more aware of what you are eating. You will have to become aware of how what you eat affects your body and how to deal with it. The problem is when something tastes that good, you tend to forget this rule of thumb.

How many times have you finished the last of something just because you didn't want it to go to waste? Or it was so good, even when you knew it was wrong, you still ate some more? Other people tend to eat as a reward and they tend to overindulge. What ever happened to eating healthier? Or eating just to live?

With the all you can eat buffets, buy one, get one free offers and dollar menus, it's hard not to overdo it every once in a while. A deal is a deal, right? The question is how do you handle it when you do overdo it?

We can't eat like we are 17, when we are in our 30s. At some point, you should know that your body is not going to react to the foods that you eat the same way that it did to what you ate when you were younger. It might not react the same way that it did a year ago. As we grow older, our bodies change to meet our age-related needs.

Think about it, in college, you probably ate pizza all the time, which is filled with carbs, but, you also probably walked a lot too. How else did you get to and from your classes? You were more active and it showed. Now, if you try that same trick, it doesn't work.

The problem with most diets again is that they always leave you feeling hungry. With some of the programs that I have tried, I felt like I was starving. Most people equate dieting with starving the body, so when you get those hunger pains, you believe that they are normal.

Like most people, when you want to want to lose a few pounds, you simply stop eating the way that you are supposed to. A meal becomes meager and in the end, you suffer both emotionally and physically because of it. You see when you starve yourself for any reason, like trying to lose weight, you are not really losing weight or that often dreaded fat, you are only losing water weight.

That's right; most of the weight that you initially lose on any diet is water weight. Water weight is brought on by years of eating the most salty foods that you can find. This is the reason why we retain so much water. This is also why most weight loss plans fail.

Most diets on this market have been designed to get rid of this water weight first. It helps to support their lies that they can help you lose 10 pounds in just one week. They rely on this by telling you to eat foods that are lower in salt, reduce your habit of adding table salt to your food and that you should start to drink more water. You could have done that on your own, without them.

Any salty food will make you thirsty. When you are thirsty, you drink more fluids and it is not always water, which is good for you. Water actually helps flush the extra salt and other toxins from your body. Anything other than just plain water, your body will hold on to it, like the empty calories in soda.

Once that water weight is gone, eventually, the body breaks down your muscle tissue to use as energy. Since you aren't eating properly. The problem is that if you had consulted your doctor first, he, or she, would have told you that, with fad dieting, you are actually doing more harm than good. You need that muscle tissue for your health's sake first.

Once the diet is over, you will find yourself falling back into your old eating habits and the water weight returns with a vengeance first. I'll explain why later, but the muscle never returns the way we need it to.

You should know that losing weight, even five pounds, has to be about changing your life and the way that you are eating, not by preventing yourself from doing it. The long term goal of any diet is for you to look better, feel better, eat better, and have more energy. That doesn't mean you have to be "thin" to do this, just healthier.

In order to change your life, you have to first change how you are living. The greatest lie that we tell ourselves is based on this belief that if we just eat less, then, ultimately, we will weigh less. Let me be the first to tell you that you are setting yourself up for a failure, one that most people never recover from, diet wise.

The key to effective weight management isn't just about how you eat. It is based on what you choose to eat, when and how much. It is also based on how active you are. When you begin to understand this, you will begin to see noticeable changes in your everyday life.

Suddenly, quality is more important than quantity in the type of foods that you are eating. Suddenly, whether or not that piece of chicken was baked or fried matters? You won't have to count calories, because you will already know what to eat and what not to eat without anyone telling you when or how to do it. It is intuitive.

You will begin to ask yourself the most important question that I have learned to ask myself before the first bite of anything that I eat, especially those barbecue potato chips that were so tempting to me last night—"Is this good for me?" If it isn't, then you shouldn't be eating it! If you are not eating what is good for you, how can you ever be good to you?

Speaking of snacks, with so many convenient snacks, how could you ever stand a fighting chance when you are trying to lose weight, you ask? It is called moderation. In plain English, don't overdo it. I recently had a pack of cookies. After eating the pack in one sitting, I finally realize that each pack came with three servings printed clearly on the bag. A serving was only three cookies, not all of them.

Everything should be done in moderation. Less of anything gives you more room to try new things, but what these diet plans and weight loss programs don't ever tell you, is that something else should always take its place. You can't suddenly stop eating white bread without learning how to replace it with whole grain bread.

Otherwise, your body begins craving what it has missed in the first place and you fall back into your old habits. We are creatures of habits. We do what we have been taught to do. It's almost comforting. Wait, it is comforting!

Eventually, many of these dieting plans and weight loss programs can also get expensive. In the end, you haven't lost weight, you have only lost valuable time and money trying to do the impossible and that is try to change the one thing that you can't--our metabolism. You can't change your metabolism! There, I said it!

I have seen one too many plans that will tell you these lies. Yes, I said it. They are lies. Any plan, that has ever, or will ever tell you, that they will help speed up your metabolism just lied to you. Tell them I said it. I'll wait.

You can't suddenly speed up your metabolism. You never could and you never will be able to. Why would you want to? What? So that you can eat like a hormonal teen-aged boy, who can eat you out of house and home and never gain a single pound.

What you might think of as your metabolism burning away those extra pounds is really hunger and your body getting ready to deal with it the only way that it knows how, by breaking down necessary muscle tissue to get the energy that it needs to survive.

The truth is that you can't speed up your metabolism any more than you can slow it down by eating a greasy cheeseburger. What you can do is to learn how to influence it. Yes, I said influence your metabolism. How? Eat more frequently. Not grazing or snacking, but eat something nourishing. Remember when I said that hungry chicks should never go hungry. That's also how you will maintain your weight loss.

Lately, there has been talk of a "metabolism fire." So start to think of your metabolism as a fire. To keep a fire going, you have to fuel it. If you run out of fuel, the fire will begin to die down. This is what happens with your metabolism, when you don't eat. The ash, once a fire burns out, is just like the fat that you store in your body and just like ash, it is hard to rekindle. Because of this the fat in your body becomes harder to remove.

You should already know that our bodies are good at storing fat. Keep this in mind when you think about what happens if you also throw too much fuel into the fire. It can go out too. If you are eating too much, that meal is hard to digest and your metabolism becomes slower as it tries to digest that heavy meal.

You will only end up storing those extra calories, instead of burning them off. That is why it is always good to eat smaller and more frequent meals throughout the day. This encourages your metabolism to keep working; like that fire does, to keep burning off the extra calories.

In the end, with any diet or weight loss plan, you should always be in control of what you eat. Not just what you eat, but how much and how often. Your goal after to every meal is to feel full, not hungry. A snack only is there to give your body energy until that next meal. Why? We will talk about that soon enough.

But, before we can get to any of that, ask yourself the one question that millions of people never ask themselves before they commit to a diet... Do I really need to lose weight? How do you know if you need to lose weight, and, if so, how much? That is one question that I must warn you that you should never ask someone that you love. Allow me to tell you why...

The Battle Of Pseudo-Obesity…

I'm certain that more fights are started in relationships by asking one question and one question alone, "Honey, do these jeans make my butt look big?" At that point, the love of your life could take things in one of two directions, they could say yes and end up sleeping on the couch or they could say no and leave you feeling vindicated, but lied to.

I would never ask my best friend either. Friends lie. Sorry, but it is the truth. I promised you that I'd tell you the truth and this is one of them. If you are going to ask your best friend if you need to lose weight, she will say that you look fine and offer you a piece of cake, if she has tried to diet too and failed. Tell her about this book.

When it comes to losing weight, there is only one person that you should ever talk to before you start any weight loss plan and that is your primary doctor, not a weight loss center counselor. Why trust your health to anyone else? You owe that much to yourself.

Ask your doctor, does he, or she, think that you need to lose weight? Especially, if there are any pressing health issues that might require you to shed a few of those extra, unwanted pounds, or an unforeseen health issue that might stop you from even trying. Either way, it is always best to ask someone who is trained to know.

The truth is most people overestimate the size of their bodies. The ideal weight, that most people see themselves at, is usually associated with a happier time in their lives, like being in college or before a pregnancy. You will find yourself thinking that if only you could get back to that weight, you will be happy again. You want to be "good" again. The greatest secret to getting back to your ideal weight is not just eating right or exercising; it is falling back in love with who you are and not with who you want to be.

Live in the moment, not the past. The problem is that often, as children, we were taught that eating all of your food equated to being "good," even when you weren't really hungry. When is overeating ever a good thing?

Right now, at this moment, you might think you are so fat, when you might just need to lose a few pounds. The problem with weight loss is in knowing how much. The real answer about this weight just might surprise you.

That's because if you are like me, you don't always see what is reflected back at you in the mirror, you often overestimate how small you are supposed to be. The truth is that many people are unaware of the fact that they might be suffering from a condition, first recognized by acclaimed author and therapist Kim Chernin, called "pseudo-obesity." Yes, pseudo-obesity. It's not real.

Pseudo-obesity is a condition, in which, many dieters may be a few pounds overweight, but to their untrained eyes, they are obese or over 20 percent of their body's ideal weight. Your ideal weight is simply the right weight for your age, height and body type.

Yet, some people are still driven nevertheless toward losing these "extra" pounds. When in reality, they should be looking to meet their ideal weight, not some unrealistic size below it.

The problem is, while most plans suggest that you attempt to lose at least 10 percent of your total body weight to feel successful. They will never tell you that this is virtually impossible if you don't need to. Instead, you should be trying to lose only one or two pounds per week until you have reached your plateau. That's the point, in your body, where your weight loss stops.

For most people, they see this plateau, or the point where their dieting efforts failed, as a frustrating period. Suddenly, no matter how hard that they have tried, they just stop losing weight. They have hit a huge road block.

You have tried to lose 30 pounds, but, can only lose 10 of those pounds. Maybe, that's all you needed to lose. The truth is that this plateau is right where you should be. It is your ideal weight determined by your body's "set points".

Most people never realize a lot of their frustration and this need to continue to lose weight is often based on an addiction to the praise that you got when people first noticed your sudden weight loss from a fad diet. It just like when somebody notices a certain color on you or a certain outfit and you keep wearing that color or that outfit to continue to get the compliments.

Fad diets depend on that rapid weight loss to keep you hooked. They know that you will then put up with whatever they tell you to, to keep using it, even if it is dangerous to your health. If that happens, you are not doing it for yourself anymore; you are doing it for other people. That is why far too many people fail at losing weight, they often get so caught up in a need to keep up with a favorite celebrity, a friend, or even, a family member's weight or weight loss. Stop trying to. Every pound that you lose is about your good health, not theirs.

That's why even after you have reached your ideal weight, you are still left with a feeling that you can never "let yourself go" again. If you do, your body will end up beyond control and you'll gain all of the weight that you lost back or that you'll gain even more weight.

This can often be the beginning of the eating disorders anorexia nervosa or bulimia. These are two conditions that you should know about before you start any weight loss effort. It's also the reason why any weight loss effort should be monitored by your doctor.

With the eating disorder known as anorexia nervosa, a person's eating habits are characterized by excessive food restriction and irrational fear of gaining weight, and a distorted body self-perception. It typically involves excessive weight loss. Anorexia nervosa usually develops during adolescence and early adulthood.

Due to the fear of gaining weight, people with this disorder restrict the amount of food that they eat. This restriction of food intake causes metabolic and hormonal disorders. The terms "anorexia nervosa" and "anorexia" are often used interchangeably; however, anorexia is simply a medical term for lack of appetite. However, people with anorexia nervosa do not lose their appetites. They simple work harder at suppressing it.

You should know that people suffering from anorexia have extremely high levels of ghrelin, the hunger hormone that tells the brain when it is time to eat, in their blood. The high levels of ghrelin suggest that their bodies are trying desperately to switch hunger on but that hunger's call is being suppressed, ignored, or overridden. This is dangerous and potentially fatal.

Bulimia nervosa is an eating disorder characterized by binge eating and purging, or consuming a large amount of food in a short amount of time, followed by an attempt to rid the body of the food consumed (purging), typically by vomiting, laxative abuse, fasting and/or excessive exercise, and commonly accompanied with fasting over an extended period of time.

Bulimia nervosa is considered to be less life threatening than anorexia; however, the occurrence of bulimia nervosa is higher and it is still very dangerous. The vast majority of those with bulimia nervosa are usually at a normal weight. The binge-purge episodes are almost always kept secret, and they tend to follow a recurring pattern with at least two episodes per week.

Like anorexia nervosa, bulimia has its roots in complex social and emotional issues and if you recognize the symptoms in you or someone that you love, you should seek immediate treatment without embarrassment. In the end, it is not what other think about you and your weight that matters, but what your doctor recommends.

With that thought in your mind, I think you are ready to get "real" about you truly losing weight. That means being honest with yourself about your weight and what you can truly afford to lose. It is time to stop listening to the ads that you see on television and in magazines about weight loss and start listening yourself…

Getting Real About Dieting And Weight Loss

Before we begin, you should know that for years, I believed every lie that I was ever told about dieting and weight loss. Yet, even in the midst of these lies, as I said before, I was still looking for a way out of the yo-yo dieting cycle; the same way a deer is looking to escape a hunter. In the end, I have learned that no new dress is worth the risk that a fad diet can place on your health.

Eventually, I began to believe my own self-doubts, "What if I can't lose this weight?" "What if I can't keep it off?" "What if I mess up?" "What happens then?" I couldn't do. What if I couldn't lose the weight that I wanted? When I did lose a few pounds, nobody ever told me how to keep it off. I was stuck.

Ask yourself what happens when life happens and that diet plan just doesn't seem to be working? What happens when your plan has worked but now, it just doesn't work anymore? How do you know when any plan has really started working properly? That's a lot of unanswered questions!

In the end, what I learned is that every doubt and all of my what-ifs, they had to be replaced by what I could do for myself. I had to get real and be honest with myself. What I said I can't do means what I won't do.

I was thinking like so many other people often do that losing weight meant burning more calories than I actually ate. The problem seemed simple, but in the end, I discovered that it wasn't. If that was the case, nobody would ever be overweight again.

Even then, when you have a car note or mortgage, buying a certain diet's meal plan next week might become an option. It might become something that you would like to do rather than something that you need to buy. Trust me, I understand, life happens.

What happens when you bought a gym membership, but, you have become too tired from every day activities to ever use it? Who has 30 minutes in our day to go for a walk? What do you do at that point? The truth is even in a world where it feels like there is never enough time in our day, we have to learn to make time.

According to the Center For Disease Control, adult obesity has become a common, costly and disturbing reality. It is estimated that that obesity, which is defined as being more than twenty percent over your ideal weight, affects more than one-third of the adults (35.7%) in the United States. That's more than 90 million Americans.

In 2011, it was determined that no state has ever met the nation's Healthy People 2010 goal to lower its obesity rate to 15%. The number of states with more than 30% of its population being obese actually rose to 12 states in 2010. In 2000, that number was zero.

What is even scarier is that it is estimated that by the year 2030, 90% of all Americans will be considered overweight. That is over 300 million people. When you stop to consider that obesity is a factor in the leading causes of death in this country, including heart disease, stroke, type 2 diabetes and certain types of cancer, this isn't something that we can afford to simply ignore. We have to get real about it.

You should know that again to really lose weight will require you to create a new reality for yourself, one that is not based on the person that you want to be, but the healthier person that you can and will be. Imagine for every dollar that you have already spent to become slimmer, the answer has been within you all along. It is based on your commitment to losing this weight.

Right now, you have a decision to make. Ask yourself how committed are you to changing the way that you eat, how much you eat and how often? That's because this goal is not an easy one. You have to enter this with a mindset that says that you will lose those extra, unwanted pounds and you are prepared to do what you have to do to keep it off. You can't do it halfheartedly.

Even then, you cannot become discouraged or afraid when your effort doesn't work right away, or the way that you wanted it to. You have to remain focused on your goal weight. Every pound that you lose is helping to create a healthier you. But, you have to be committed to this plan. Again, your commitment is the key to making this work. Losing weight takes commitment.

Your ultimate goal is not to be a size two, but maybe be a healthy size eight. You won't wake up one day and look like Angelina Jolie, but you can wake up being a 20 pound lighter version of you, 20 pounds that could mean the difference between a heart attack, or having a longer, healthier life. You have a decision to make.

If the motivation and desire to grow healthier has never been this strong within you, the problem is not that you haven't gotten truly real about what to expect from any diet plan. You just have never been realistic about what you can lose in weight and what you can gain when it comes to your life. It is about more than being thin.

You have to say to yourself, this is what I want and make it happen for yourself. Say it aloud if you can right now, "I want to look better. I want to feel better. I want to eat better. I want to have more energy."

Say this when you wake up in the morning. Say it to yourself in the shower. Say this as you travel to work. Say it as you walk, jog or run. You'll need it. Often the best advice that anyone can give is what we tell ourselves. If we believe it, we can, then, achieve it.

The one thing that you can't do is depend on a diet or anything that is labeled low fat or reduced calories to do all of the work for you. You can't eat anything that you want, but, you can still enjoy the foods that you love without guilt. The key again is moderation.

In the end, your decision to lose weight is not about how well you will fit into those old pair of jeans or that new dress. It is about you. Given time, you will see results that you never thought could be possible. But, a change can only come when your decision to eat healthier becomes something that you want to do and not something that you only think that you should do.

I should warn you though that the problem has never been just about your determination to lose weight. It also isn't just about how honest many of these plans have been with you either. The problem might be how honest you are being with yourself about how "thin" you will be and what really goes into maintaining your weight loss. You can't just lose the weight, and then, go back to eating how you used to and not working out.

Fantasy about losing weight may be what you want, but a dose of reality is what you need. It is time to retire from the fantasy that says you need to be a size two to be healthy. Stop allowing the media to determine what your weight should be. Stop comparing your body to other people, they are not you. All body types are beautiful and you should love everything about yours.

To be healthy, you might only need to lose five or ten pounds to return to your ideal weight. The trick is in finding out what that is. I am going to show you. Once you do know, then, I am going to show you the most proven and effective way to help you lose that weight and how to finally reach your ideal weight or goal weight.

Being real is not about being as thin as you can get; being real means understanding what you can and cannot do when it comes to finding your ideal weight and reaching it. If you didn't notice, for the last couple of chapters, not once have I told you how skinny you should be. It has all about being healthier. Good health brings weight loss and better weight management.

The truth is not everyone was born to be a size two. I am being very honest with you. You should know that that's because there is something else in your DNA that is making it virtually impossible to ever get there. I mentioned it before, it is called a "set point" and I think that it's about time that we talk about it...

Not Every One Was Meant To Be A Size Two...

If being a size 12 is a constant struggle, what if I told you that that struggle is the first warning sign of being overweight? Your true size, or ideal weight, is the size that your body feels most comfortable at. The problem is that very few people actually adhere to what their bodies tell them to do. When they are hungry, they don't eat. When they are full, they don't stop eating.

What if I told you that you are born to be a certain size? Deep down in your DNA, there is a genetic code that determined everything at your birth, from what color your eyes were going to be to the height that you are right now. What if this code also predicted your weight?

This explains why you have that one thin friend, who can eat as much as she want and never gain any weight. But, you are always hungry and everything that you eat spends a moment on your lips and a lifetime on your hips. That's because you are not her.

You see these genetic codes create in the body, what health officials call "set points." If your current weight loss plan didn't tell you this, stop using them right away. You probably already have. They are setting you up for failure. Look at Oprah, she is probably now at her set point, after years of struggling with her weight.

What a set point does in the body is to determine how much weight your body can maintain without any effort. It is sort of like breathing. It is something that happens if we think about it or not. This should be your goal weight.

If, at any point, our bodies go below that point, our bodies react in a ruthless way to return us back to our "normal weight." You will feel sluggish and tired. You will also always feel very hungry. It sort of the same way that a car begins to act when it is running out of gas.

Starvation mode, more formally known as famine response, is part of your body's survival system. When you aren't eating enough nutritious foods, your body will, then, fall into a famine response mode. That's because normally, when a person isn't eating enough. Your body thinks that there isn't any food to eat. This starvation mode will slow down the body's metabolism to try and save as much energy as it can.

According to the study, "The Biology of Human Starvation" from the University of Minnesota Press, Starvation mode kicks in after three days of continuous fasting, when you haven't eaten properly, or when you have lowered the amount of calories that you usually eat, i.e. you are dieting. You already know those feelings of hunger and how horrible they can be. That's your body's way of saying, "Eat something!"

You should also know that your body also sends these hunger signals, i.e. that growling stomach, when you are tired, dehydrated or feeling psychological hunger. If you use what I am going to teach you, you should never feel like this. Hungry chicks should go feel hungry!

Wait! What is psychological hunger, you asked? Psychological hunger, or rebound hunger, is when we still feel hungry even after a full meal. That's because your body hasn't told your brain that you are full or you just might be craving a specific food, like you are craving potato chips or chocolates. At that point, drink some cold water and let the feeling pass.

When your body is telling you to eat, it believes there is still food to be eaten, so there is no starvation mode yet. When you continue to not eat properly, usually after about 3 to 5 days, your body has decided that there must not be any food and uses alternative energy sources, like breaking down your muscle tissue. Then, your body will again work to conserve your energy.

That's the reason why starvation diets can cause up to a 50 percent muscle loss. That's because your body is getting rid of something that uses a lot of energy and because it needs the protein that your muscle provides, when it breaks down that muscle tissue.

That's because your body is simply not getting enough protein when you are only eating small amounts of food, or no food at all. Our muscle tissue will provide the same protein found in lean meats that our body needs. That's why eating lean meat and other sources of protein are essential to our good health.

That's also why some women end up looking like skin and bones after some extreme dieting. Their bodies have already rid itself of necessary muscle tissue. Not fat, necessary muscle tissue.

You will again feel tired and sluggish. This is your body's way of conserving energy so that you will rest. It will also boost your appetite to the point where you will find yourself eventually eating anything and everything when this "fasting" stops. You are hungry and your body will do everything in its power to get what it needs.

For instance, let's say that you went on a crash diet for six weeks in order to get ready for a class reunion, or even, a wedding. You might have gone without eating a regular meal for weeks. You might have skipped breakfast, substituted lunch with a snack, and then, you ate a light dinner. You were basically starving yourself. You should have been hungrier than ever before.

In order to protect itself, your body goes into this starvation mode and in order to survive, your body increased its capabilities to store more fat. Where does this fat come from? The truth is anything that you eat. Just look at the labels. The problem is your body doesn't care if it is good fat or bad fat. The body will do anything to survive. Anything? Anything!

This too is in our DNA, it comes from a time when our ancestors often had to migrate to find food, so they tended to splurge when they could find food and this helped during the lean times when food was not always plentiful as it is now. They basically fasted.

What does this mean for you? It means that it will be nothing, once you return to your old eating habits, to find yourself weighing more than you first began your diet. In essence, dieting can actually make you more overweight than you could ever believe by hoarding fat. That's because your body is fighting to survive. It doesn't care that you want to be a smaller size again.

The other issue that most diet plans and programs fail to deal with is the psychological difficulties of trying to lose weight. No, you are not crazy and never will be. But, you might recognize some of the signs of what health officials call "dieting depression syndrome." Dieting depression syndrome causes those feelings of irritability, anxiety, depression, mood swings and fatigue that you feel while dieting. This syndrome is very real.

On some diets, you tend to become overly sensitive to stress that can result from that diet, especially when that highly restrictive diet forces you to stop eating many of the foods that you love to achieve a certain weight loss. You might even find yourself turning to food to relieve this stress. Don't do it. This is a huge mistake.

Stop and thinking about why you to quit your last diet. What was the reason that you quit? A cookie? You already know how it feels when a cookie, stops being a cookie and becomes a source of comfort. Not only do you find comfort for the stress, that you are feeling, just by eating it, but you will find that you have chosen one of the most sugar-laden foods available.

These "treats" are capable of increasing the mood elevating chemicals in your brain, the same way a mood altering drug does. Yes, a cookie can do that for you. The less that you are allowed to eat, the more tempting that even a cookie will look to you. This is why you should never restrict any foods from your diet, unless you necessarily have to for health reasons or you find out that it is bad for you. For anything else, again, take into consideration, moderation.

Now that I have told you about how to get real about your ideal weight, I will bet you that nobody has ever told you how to find your ideal or goal weight. That is until now. How about it has been as close as your wrist all of this time and you didn't even know it...

Determining Your Ideal Or Goal Weight...

While most dieting efforts will tell you about some complicated way to determine your idea weight, I kept thinking that there has to be a simpler way. You don't even want to know what I was thinking when I heard about the BMR chart at first. That's when I discovered something that changed my life.

I found a better way to determine my ideal weight. You see most people fall into three categories. Either you have a small frame, a medium frame or a large frame. The following chart is the best way to tell which one you are, so that you can determine your ideal weight.

Here's how it works...let's say that you are a woman that has a wrist size of 5 ¾ inches, which indicates a medium frame. You currently weigh 150 pounds, but you are only five feet four inches. Upon checking the chart, you discover that your idea weight should be between 124 and 138 pounds. You could benefit from losing about 15 to 20 pounds. Pretty simple, huh? It is!

To find yours, first measure the circumference, or the distance around your wrist. For women, 5 ½ inches or less means a small frame, 5 ½ to 6 ¼ inches indicates a medium frame and anything over 6 ¼ is a large frame.

Let's take a moment to determine your ideal weight, for your body, using this chart. For example, 5' 2" means 5 feet two inches. This number is now your goal for your ideal body weight. Remember this. Write it down.

Remember that an ideal weight it just that, it is ideal. It is an indicator of where we would like to be. This is your weight loss goal or where you can be. When setting goals like this, how specific have you been?

Goals should be SMART. Your goal should be specific, measurable, attainable, relevant and time bound. For example, you should say, "I can and will lose 10 pounds, or about a pound a week, within the next three months. Specific: lose weight. Measurable: 10 pounds. Attainable: a pound a week. Time bound: Within in three months, which is 12 weeks, which gives you room to breathe and time to start over, if you make a mistake.

Ideal Weights For Women

Your Height	Small Frame	Medium Frame	Large Frame
4' 10"	102-11	109-121	118-131
4' 11"	103-113	111-123	120-134
5' 0"	104-115	123-126	122-137
5' 1"	106-121	115-129	125-140
5' 2"	108-121	118-132	128-143
5' 3"	111-124	121-135	131-147
5' 4"	114-127	124-138	134-151
5' 5"	117-130	127-141	137-155
5' 6"	120-133	130-144	140-159

5' 7"	123-136	133-147	143-163
5' 8"	126-139	136-150	146-167
5' 9"	129-139	139-153	149-170
5' 10"	132-145	142-156	152-173
5' 11"	135-148	145-159	155-176
6' 0"	138-151	148-162	158-179

What is your ideal weight? Did you write your ideal weigh down! Do it now, before you forget! This is your new weight loss goal! Now, say it aloud...

...I will be _____ pounds.

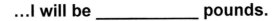

Now that you have figured out your ideal weight, the next thing that you now have to do is to come to grips with is the most destructive relationship that you have ever had. No, it is not with your parents, or even a past relationship. You will only wish that it was that simple.

You should know that when you are overweight, the most destructive relationship in your life has been with food. Yes, food. If you thought that a personal relationship was hard enough, then, your relationship with food, yes, food, surely hasn't been a picnic. The worst part is that you already knew this...

Understanding Your Relationship With Food

Have you ever thought about the relationship that you have with food? The truth is that this just might be the most intimate, yet destructive relationship that you have ever had in your life. This relationship hasn't always been a very good one. We often spend more time with food than we spend with our own families.

On the surface, food is a necessity. It is as essential as the air that we breathe. But for millions of people, food has taken on another role. Some people eat to live and some live to eat, which only makes it that much harder to build a healthy relationship with food and allow it to become something that we should enjoy. Many people treat it like another chore. That's why so many people hate to cook, but, they love to eat.

The problem is that this volatile relationship didn't start recently. It started in our childhood. I mentioned "being good." Growing up, at some point, all of us have been told that if we don't finish our food that we won't get dessert. Or that if we didn't finish our food, we weren't even allowed to leave the table. How many times did we scarf food down our throats just to get back outside, so that we can play some more? Probably, all of us.

It is at that point that food then took on a personal relationship for many of us. If we ate all of our food, it was a sign of "being good." What started out as a necessity became a symbol of our well being. A clean plate often made you feel better about yourself temporarily. Why should you have to rely on a clean plate to tell you that you are full and to stop eating?

Most of us still haven't forgotten the old wives' tale that our mothers used to tell us when we sat at the table and played with your food. It was always the same story that we shouldn't play with our food when there are people in China, who were starving. She always went on to say how much they would love to eat what I had for dinner.

Even as a child, that never stopped me from wondering to myself, how did my mother even know about those people when she had never even been to China? Of course, I didn't have the nerve to even dare to ask her that, so I cleaned my plate. I wanted to be good. I also wanted the chance to eat my dessert, even if I was full.

Since then, food has become a symbol of everything that is good about our lives. What is New Year's Eve without a party? Valentine's Day must be chocolate's best friend. On Saint Patrick's Day, sure I'll have some wings with a pint of green beer. Easter meant dinner at your grandmother's and you knew that the food was going to be good, right down to the mashed potatoes.

Mother's Day isn't Mother's Day without Mom being treated to breakfast, in bed or at her favorite restaurant. Memorial's Day...barbecue anyone? Father's Day, Dad gets to pick where we eat. Fourth of July...did someone say barbecue? Summer pool parties...burgers and hot dogs. Yes! Yum. Yum. Labor Day...did you want a hamburger or a hot dog? Who said tailgate party?

Halloween...ooh, candy! Thanksgiving is all about the drumstick and the mashed potatoes. Christmas is all about Mom's ham. Let's not forget everything in between. Bill in accounting is retiring, let's have cake! It's my birthday—cake! Your nephew turned three—

cake! Date night isn't date night without dessert. Super bowl Sunday, who ordered wings? You get my point!

The problem is that we use food for all of the wrong reasons. We turn to food for comfort when we are sad, depressed, hurt, or even, angry. A carton of ice cream is often your best friend. The sugar rush is enough to often elevate our mood and our spirit, the problem is that it will also increase our waist lines.

How many times have you met friends for coffee, but it turns into a full blown lunch? I can go through a bucket of popcorn just watching a movie and I won't even realize it until my hand reaches the bottom of the bucket. We even eat when we are bored. Yes, bored!

The real problem is when food becomes an addiction and, with 24 hour food channels, an obsession. Restaurants know this and supermarkets thrive on this. Their goal is to prey on your weakness and to get you to spend even more money.

It doesn't help you when a store asks for your zip code. They are targeting you for their advertising. What is even scarier is how effective that some of this advertising is. They know how to keep their commercials in your head, so do food companies.

Ask yourself how Tony the Tiger is? Great, right? What sounds do Rice Krispies make? If you can finish this sentence, "Time to make the _____." I rest my case. The answer is donuts, as in, Dunkin Donuts. Yet, you pause when someone asked you for your phone number. You will say that you don't call yourself. So, you don't remember it. But, it's your phone number.

How on earth can you forget that? But, you know that food jingle!

In our relationship with food, we have been taught that the answer to any problem is food. I love the Golden Girls reruns just like the next person. Those ladies loved to eat! So, it's no surprise whenever one of the ladies had a problem, they solved it over a cheese cake.

We ultimately forget that food, along with shelter, clothing and love are the cornerstones to our very existence. Because of this, our relationship with food becomes that much more complicated. Right now, let me show you why even that doesn't have to be.

Let's start over and begin to look at food in a new light. In order to better handle your commitment to looking better, feeling better, eating better and gaining more energy, you have to learn how to recognize what is triggering you eat. Are you eating because you are hungry or are you eating just to eat? Awareness is key! Awareness is what brings about change!

Second, you must change your habits. You can no longer say that you're eating out of boredom or habit. You must find other ways to occupy your time. It might be a walk, a talk, or even, a nap. If your relationship with other people is based on your on food, take the food portion out of it. Go for a walk, instead of lunch.

Sure, you might not be able to escape pasta night at your parents', but you don't have to eat it all in one sitting. On a date night, eat before the movie, or find another way to socialize without food. If that is not possible, let's develop a goal of moderation. Too much of anything is, well, too much.

What I always encourage when trying anything new is what I call a "no thank you bite." It allows you to try just about anything without overdoing it. You don't have to say, I'll have a "no thank you bite," which is what samples in a store usually are. You can say that you'll try it, but only ask for a little bit or a smaller piece.

Moderation, in the form of a "no thank you bite," or you simply telling your host that you will just have a small piece of something, allows you to enjoy it without hurting anyone's feelings. By denying yourself, you are only setting yourself up for failure the next time that you are in the same position or facing a severe craving.

This allows you to remain in control of what you are eating. One of the biggest issues in losing weight is also not thinking about what you eat and losing that control over what and how much you eat. Weight management is always about what you eat, how much and how often.

Again, ask yourself, "Is this good for me?" If it isn't, then why are you eating it? If I am not eating something that is good for me, then, I am not being good to me.

Right now, you should know that I'd never forgive myself if I didn't also talk about the where when it comes to your relationship with food. Where you eat tends to be just as important as the "what" you eat. This is another key to losing weight.

When I eat anything, I also try to sit at a table and eat off a plate. It forces me to be aware of my surroundings and what I am eating. Eating on the run is tempting, but, no real thought goes in to it. It becomes something that you just do. It also becomes a poor eating habit. That's why I also try not to eat in the living room in front of the television or in my bedroom.

I also have a rule that I try to stick to and that is to turn off and tune in. When you are sitting in front of a television, or talking on the phone, it is easy to lose track of what you are eating and how much. You aren't even looking at your food. You also run the risk of not even tasting what you have just eaten. How can you? It's already gone. Learn to savor the flavor of your food.

Part of the reason why it is so easy for many people to gain weight is because they don't even chew their food the proper number of times, they merely swallow it. How many times have you done this as a child?

If you stop and think about it, you have been doing it now for years, as an adult, during your own 30 minute lunch and you feel bad about it later on. Every office usually comes with a lunchroom or break area, bring your lunch and use it. Old habits die hard, but some were meant to be broken, like rushing through a meal.

This brings me back to what I meant about food being one of the most destructive relationships that you ever had. How else can you explain why people tend to be angry with themselves over something that they have told themselves that they shouldn't have eaten? Why should a bag of chips make you feel guilty?

Think about the last time that you splurged and ordered the chocolate sundae for dessert? The first thing you probably said before you even ordered it was that you shouldn't have. But you did and you felt guilty about it. Your stomach wasn't upset by the sundae, you were upset and that is why your stomach was upset. Every food has the potential to be bad for you, because of fat, calories, carbs or even what it is made of. You just have to learn how to exercise moderation with any food that you eat.

If you are out with your family at the beach and the best food that you can get is French fries, don't berate yourself for eating them! Eat them. Just make a healthier choice the next time that hunger strikes, if you can. It also doesn't mean that you skip dinner because you ate those fries. You will only pay for that later on.

Also, give up the all or nothing attitude that says that if you don't finish that sandwich, nobody else can. Unless you are under 18 and have to live by your parents' rules, learn to eat when you are hungry and stop when you are full. Eat some now and save some for later. If you are eating with someone, don't be afraid to share it.

Eat only when you are hungry and stop when you are full. If you deny yourself food, you most likely will overeat when you finally do eat. Your stomach is only the size of your fist and it tends to fill up rather quickly. When you allow yourself to get but so hungry, you will soon learn that your body will not stop until it is satisfied, not when you feel satisfied by what you have eaten.

It is also okay not to finish everything. Wrap it up and save it for later. Really, it's okay. Sometimes, last night's dinner leftovers will make a great lunch the next day. I know. I have had leftovers from dinner at lunch the next day. It is delicious, especially when the seasonings have had a chance to marinate. Maybe, that's why most foods have always tasted better the next day.

By understanding your relationship with food, you will spend less time thinking about it. The less time that you spend thinking about it will end a lot of unnecessary cravings. This will also save you a lot of time, money and pounds from your late night binges, giving you a chance to eat better, weigh less and become healthier.

Every time that you even think about going into your kitchen, ask yourself this question, "Am I even hungry?" In many cases, the answer just might surprise you. You might not be hungry at all. You might just be thirsty.

Again, try drinking a glass of cold water and wait about 20 minutes. If you still feel hungry, then eat something, if not relax. Your body just confused thirst with hunger. You should always drink something before you eat anything anyway. I'll tell you why soon enough.

Now that we have talked about your relationship with food, let's talk about how to shop without temptations holding you back, Shopping should always be treated like seeing that ex-boyfriend, yes, him, who you were once crazy about and maybe, even in love with.

Now, when you see him, you don't feel the same way about him that you once did. When you walk away, you actually feel better without him. Let's try that with some of the most tempting foods in the supermarket. Again, supermarkets thrive off of your destructive relationship with food and it is costing you your waist line...

How To Shop Your Supermarket Smarter

Smart shopping takes planning and requires a lot of effort on your part. Every year people waste 160 billion pounds of food. Food that could have gone to feed the millions of families that will go hungry in this country and around the world every day. When you are struggling to put food on the table, every last piece of bread counts.

With the average family, you should know most of the food in our homes often goes to waste because our cabinets and refrigerators are often packed with food. A lot of this is food that we don't eat, don't need or don't want. We buy it out of habit or because it is on sale, rather than a real desire to eat it.

You might want to cook a pot roast recipe that you saw on Rachel Ray. You bought all of the ingredients, but out of convenience, that night you ate at McDonald's instead. Thanks, Ronald!

There is even a local market in Philadelphia that is open 24 hours a day. Many stores are now open 24 hours a day. This is a foodie's dream! I can get a pint of ice cream and a cake at three in the morning!

These markets offer some of the best produce, the best cakes, and even, a hot bar with freshly made foods. It also makes more than a million dollar every week. Grocery stores aren't designed to help you eat better. It is places like this that helps you understand why your mother always said to always make a list before you go.

Supermarkets again thrive on your destructive relationship with food. Every part of the market is designed to make you spend more money and buy more food than you really need. Given how much food we waste, ask yourself how much food do you even eat every year? Remember how much food you waste?

But, I digress; let's take a trip to the market. Let's say that you were running low on milk and bread. Ask yourself then why is your cart filled with everything from the ice cream that was on sale to the donuts that smelled so good when you walked by?

Oh, the soup was on sale too. Okay! No, judgment here. You also brought that magazine because Ryan Reynolds was on the cover. At least, it's not food. Don't eat anything while you read it. Have you ever been in the market, was reading a magazine in the checkout lane and subconsciously opened a bag of chips because you were so engrossed in a one of the articles? I know that I have.

Now, I also tend to shy away from the processed meats from the deli department at my favorite supermarket. Why? That's because a few feet away is the bakery section. As I am standing in line waiting for my cold cuts, I am tempted to buy another cake to see if my powder sugar trick really works.

The first five times, I was skeptical, but this time, I might work my magic. Maybe, I wasn't using the right "fairy dust" or powder sugar, if you must, on it. Don't judge me. I was trying to do what that woman said to do.

Now, when I smell any cake, my salivary glands really get going. The smell of a bakery is like second hand smoke, it should be illegal. Stores know this, that's why you always can smell the fresh baked goods from anywhere in the store. So now, I am now hungry and more inclined to buy a lot of other things that I really don't need. Maybe, that's why my mother also said never to go to the supermarket hungry either.

Wait, you came for milk too. That is in the back of the store, which requires you to walk all the way through the store to get to it. Since you got milk, why not get a pack of Oreos to go with it. Wait, you should see what else is on sale. Let's grab a circular. Ten TV dinners, that usually cost 99 cents, are on sale for ten dollars.

Wait, you did need to get more cereal, right? Good thing the store thought ahead and made it convenient for you to buy the most expensive cereals by placing them at eye level and within your reach. Thanks!

Did you know you tend to buy more of any item that is on the right hand side of the aisle? You do now. That's where the most expensive items are. But, then again, when you go to the market, everything that is on your right hand side. If you try to move your cart to the left it is hard to do. There is even a disabling device on the cart, if you take the cart too far away from the market.

Don't ever take your children to the market with you, because everything they want is at their eye level and brightly colored to grab their attention! Size also does matter. If a store is larger, even when it's crowded; it allows people to continue to impulse buy, even kids.

Wait! Do you hear that? Slow music often makes people take their time. Loud music helps keep the traffic moving and when the store plays classical music, people tend to buy more expensive items.

As you stand in the checkout line, you know you want those jelly beans, wait until I tell you what's in them. Oh, you already have two in the cart. Okay, checkout. Oh, you didn't save anything? That's okay; the store now knows what you might want to buy the next time.

Stop and think about it, yes, even those nice coupons that they print out with your receipt are about you. They are based on your past purchases, will expire even sooner to get you to buy more items faster, which means that you will spend even more money. How? They make you feel like you are actually saving money. The truth is you aren't. You're spending more money.

I have learned to go to the market only once a week. Second, I always make a list of what I need and I try to come up with a budget that I can stick to. If I still have eggs. I won't buy more, just in case. I buy what I eat.

Before I go, I will have a light snack; this keeps me from impulse buying to suit a craving. I buy only what I need, when I need it. This strategy will save you valuable time and money too. You can't eat what you don't buy.

The key again is to make a shopping list, based on what you want to eat for the week. You can take a simple calendar and write out a list of the meals that you want and it will consist of the things that you will need to make it. Saturday might be chicken, Sunday fish.

If I freeze what I buy, I tend to season or cook it before I do. If it is already seasoned, I can set it out to thaw out before I leave for work and pop it into the oven when I get home. If it is already cooked, I can just pop it in the microwave and it can be ready to eat in about the same amount of time that it will take me to order Chinese takeout or a pizza. Spaghetti sauce is the best. All you have to do is boil the pasta to have it for lunch or dinner.

When you do shop, focus on the heart healthy items, like low fat milk, low fat cheese and lean pieces of meat. Since dairy, meat, bakery and vegetables are on the perimeter, or the walls of the store, I shop the interior with care. When in doubt of how good something is for me, I check the label out. Always shop just like you should eat, with calories, fat and salt in mind, as you do.

The interior is filled with processed foods that have added sugar, fat and a lower nutritional value. Whenever possible, I try to fill my cart with as few processed foods as possible. Some of your favorite foods are already loaded with salt.

The lower the salt that you consume, the more water weight that you will lose and not muscle. Most Americans get about 3,400 milligrams of sodium in their daily diets, according to Mayo Clinic, a non-profit medical practice and medical research group based in Minnesota, that specializes in treating the most difficult cases, including weight loss. That's too much salt!

The daily recommended intake for adults under age 50 is 2,300 milligrams per day, which is roughly 1.5 tablespoons. If you are age 51 or older, you should be getting about 1,500 milligrams per day or less. Keep in mind, that these are upper limits for all salt and sodium.

Eating less salt is always best, whenever possible and better for your health. You owe that much to yourself.

As you shop, the best way to avoid excessive sodium or salt servings is to buy foods labeled only "low sodium," "very low sodium" or "sodium free." Low sodium foods contain less than 140 milligrams of sodium per serving while very low sodium foods have less than 35 milligrams of sodium per serving. This is better for you.

Sodium-free foods have less than 5 milligrams per serving. If you stick to eating these types of foods, you can keep your sodium intake per serving relatively low. Also, pay careful attention to the serving sizes. A low-sodium food can quickly become high in sodium if you eat more than the recommended serving size.

Extra salt causes extra weight. Eventually, you will reach a point in your life where your body will know when something is too salty and you can drink extra water to help flush the extra salt out of your system. You can no longer depend on luck to help you lose weight. Nor can you wish it away. Yet, there is something that you can buy to help you...fresh or low sodium foods.

So what's next? Now that you understand what didn't work before in your dieting, why these plans have been designed to fail, you have an idea of where you would like to be in your weight loss goals, you know how to shop and are beginning to understand your relationship with food. The next step requires a simple phone call...

The One Thing That Only Your Doctor Could Or Should Know About You...

The next step in all of this is to get a physical! That's right, a complete physical. A physical actually tells your doctor if there are any health issues that might be causing your weight gain or hindering your weight loss.

If you have ever tried and failed at a diet, there might be a serious medical reason why you have failed. Trying to lose weight is often a relentless cycle for many people. That's also you should always tell your doctor about your dieting successes, and even, your dieting failures.

Years of bad choices, or bad habits, that you made in what you eat and how you eat, aren't always the reason why you can't lose weight. There might be another medical reason for your weight gain, one that only your doctor could and should know. Find out what that is.

This physical should include having your weight and blood pressure checked, and then, some blood work done to check for any blood disorders, such as anemia. You should also have your blood sugar checked for diabetes, making this blood work very important.

This blood work will also allow you to check on your thyroid, which produces the hormones that affect your metabolism. When your thyroid doesn't work, it could cause weight gain among other problems. Also, be sure to get your cholesterol levels checked.

Also, ask about the medications that you are taking. If you have never read all of the side effects of some drugs that you might have been prescribed in the past, you might have overlooked that many of them cause weight gain. Did you know that certain diabetic medications, steroids, anti-depressants, high blood pressure and anti-seizure medicines can cause weight gain? It might even be caused by an over the counter medicine and you didn't even know it.

There are now over 100 drugs on the market that can cause weight gain. If you have tried to lose weight and can't or you are steadily gaining weight, you need to let your doctor know. An honest conversation with your doctor will help him, or her, to figure out how to help you.

The problem with even that is that very few people are willing to talk to their doctor about something like this until it is too late. If my doctor prescribes me anything, the first question that I ask is "Is this going to have any negative side effects, and if so, how should I deal with it?" I don't want to take anything that is going to hurt me. If your doctor doesn't bring it up, then, you should do it.

There is also another reason why you should be candid with your doctor—it increases your likelihood to stick with this dieting solution by knowing what the risks are if you don't. You can only learn about this risk from somebody who is trained to know, not a weight loss center counselor, who is paid to pretend to know what only your doctor could and should already know.

Once you have had your physical, you will be in a better position to decide what you should do next, until then, let's talk about what you can do now. Let's talk about portions and how much is really enough...

When It Comes To Portions, Know What's Fair

Most diets will often tell you what you can and cannot eat. Most don't always tell you exactly how much you can eat. I am here to tell you what is right and what is fair to you. The goal is to not just to lose weight, but to also fight those ever present hunger pains

The biggest secret to eating healthier is that anything that you eat should only be slightly bigger than your fist. Your first is actually about the size of your stomach. You don't need a calorie counter to remember this rule.

That piece of cake might look good, but is it bigger than your fist? That piece of chicken, if it is bigger than your fist, then chances are you won't be able to finish it. It is just too much. Don't even try to finish it all.

The only time that you can break this rule is when you are eating fruits and vegetables. For any vegetable, the brighter the color, or the darker it is, like broccoli or spinach, the better it is for you. That's because it has more vitamins and nutrients that your body really needs.

Using a smaller plate also helps with this rule. If it can't fit on your plate, then it's too much. The problem with that is most people tend to pile food on top of food. They figure that since it is all going down the same way, why not? Break this habit right away.

Spread your food out, if you can't see it, then, you shouldn't eat it and you won't be able to savor the flavor of it. This is very important. Savoring food means eating slower and actually taking the time to enjoy it.

According to the American Institute For Cancer Research, portion sizes in America have grown too large. You should aim for meals that are made up of two-thirds (or more) of vegetables, fruits, whole grains or beans and only one-third of animal based protein (meat). This will allow you gradually transition from the old American plate that looked like this...

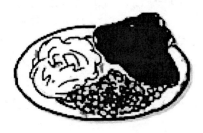

To a better plate that looks something like this...

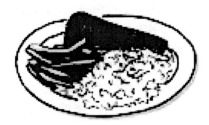

To what your new American plate should look like.

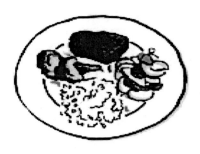

To make your meal more appealing, it helps to use health oils like olive oil, canola oil and fruit juice for cooking, on salads, and at the table. Limit any butter and trans fats, which can be found in cooking oils, in your diet. If it seems like I am repeating this message, I am. I want you to learn it, and then, use it.

The more vegetables on your plate, the better things will be for you and the more variety, the better. Anything made with a potato, which is a starch doesn't count. As mentioned before, the brighter the color of the fruit or vegetable the better that it is for you. You just have to find out what you might like, and then, eat more of it.

During the meal, also try to drink as much water as possible. There is a reason why they put water on the table at a restaurant. It not only helps clean your palate, but, allows you to really taste every part of your meal. It also gives you a better chance to feel fuller quicker. If you drink water before you eat, it helps your digestion.

Avoid sugary drinks at dinner time. Limit milk to 1 or 2 glasses a day. Limit even juices to one glass a day. If you have a sugar craving, try eating a piece of fruit for dessert. Add brown rice, whole grain pasta and breads, like honey wheat, to your meal. Honey wheat is actually delicious. Limit refined grains, like white rice and white bread. This refining often removes all of the nutrients.

When it comes to protein, choose fish, poultry, beans and nuts. Limit red meat to lean cuts like flank, chuck or sirloin steak and to less than eight ounces per meal. Limit cold cuts, fatty bacon and other processed meats.

Never put any serving bowls on the table. This is the number one reason why most people splurge at dinner. It makes things that much more tempting when it comes to having seconds. It is right there with no additional effort needed, enabling you to overdo it.

Also, when there is too much food, don't force yourself to finish it. You are no longer a member of the clean plate club. When in doubt, eat half. If your favorite restaurant gives away a lot of food, save some for later. When in doubt, try to do what children do--don't eat it.

Did you know why most children are often the best at maintaining their weight? They are active thanks to recess and afternoon play time. More importantly, when a child tells you that they are not hungry, believe them. Nine times out of ten, it's because unlike you, they have been eating all day. Here is why...

When a child, maybe your child, wakes up, they tend to eat breakfast. The public school systems even offer it. You might even pack them a snack to eat at recess. It might be something as simple as a granola bar, but it helps. Then, they eat lunch. At lunch, they often share what they have with their friends when it is too much.

After school, you, or their afterschool programs, often provides them with a nutritious snack. So by the time that they eat dinner, they may not be hungry or only eat very little before declaring that they are full. Many parents are upset about this. They think that their child is supposed to eat, but really the child is smarter. Children only eat when they want to, not because they have to. What about you? What do you do?

You may forget all about eating until your appointed time and when you do, often it is too late. You aren't feeling sluggish at two in the afternoon because you are overworked; you are tired because your body wasn't properly fed. Instead of taking a snack break, most people will go smoke a cigarette.

Snacks are also important for you. They don't have to be a full blown meal; a snack can be as simple as a bag of almonds or peanuts that you keep on your desk. It will give you a nice boast of energy, without the calories of a bag of barbecue potato chips or some greasy fries. You just need a hand full laid out flat on your palm.

When spread flat on your palm, that equals about one ounce of nuts. Your palm is also the size of three ounces of meat. This will help when you are thinking about calories, but don't have this book to fall back on.

Here are a few other quick measuring tips that might help you. Did you know that your fist is also the size of one cup of rice, cereal or oatmeal? The size of your finger tip is about one half teaspoon of olive oil. Two fingers are about an ounce of cheese. It is so simple.

Try also using the same trick that our parents used on us. When we were younger, they figured our stomachs and our mouths were smaller, so they cut our food up. Did you know that this creates an optical illusion for our minds? That same bagel that you ate this morning, cut up would have made you feel fuller, faster, just by cutting it into four pieces before you ate it?

I also realized that my mother was right; you really should chew your food about 30 times. Not only does it help your digestion, but it gives your stomach time to send a signal to your brain to say that you are full. Then, learn to rest your fork between bites; give yourself time to chew what you already have in your mouth.

Also, when you are eating anything, again, pay attention to the serving sizes. A bag of cookies might have two or three servings in it. Become aware of them. Then, if you need to, share them like children do. If you are hungry enough to eat the whole bag, then, you are not eating enough of the foods that are good for you.

How much you put at the end of your fork is just as powerful as what you put at the end of your fork. Food is an information source for your body. Your body depends on it to tell it what to do. If you do eat too much, your body will become confused by this.

If you don't eat enough, your body doesn't know what to do. When you eat the right amount, your body will know exactly what to do, when and how. Food is power, use this power to help you lose weight and keep it off.

Speaking of when, if time is an issue for you during the day, try preparing your lunch the night before. This allows you to know what you are eating and removes the temptation to splurge on a bunch of processed foods, like a hot dog from a local vendor's cart.

Wait, I'll bet nobody ever told you what was in that hot dog. Sure, it might be America's favorite food, but will it be yours after what I tell you? I think it is only fair that I tell you what else is in it, besides a lot of salt…

Think It's Only A Hot Dog? Let Me Be Frank...

According to the National Hot Dog and Sausage Council, "All hot dogs are cured and cooked sausages that consist of mainly pork, beef, chicken and turkey or a combination of those meats and poultry.

Meats used in hot dogs come from the muscle of the animal and looks much like what you buy in the grocer's case." Contrary to popular belief, it is not made up chicken heads and leftover meat. "Other ingredients include water, curing agents and spices, such as garlic, salt, sugar, ground mustard, nutmeg, coriander and white pepper."

However, there are a couple of other things that you should know. For instance, if these hot dogs were bought in a store, they are encased in a natural, or possibly synthetic, collagen casing. Yes, the same collagen used in beauty treatments to gain fuller lips or reduce frown lines in your face. Sounds gross right?

Natural collagen casings are a type of casing that is made to be eaten with a sausage. It is made of beef hides. The beef hides have had the hair removed, and then, the skins are rolled into thin sheets. From these sheets, tubes are formed to hold the sausage material.

Sheep intestine casings are used for small, lightweight sausages, such as breakfast links. Hog intestine casings are the most popular size as they are used for traditional sausage rolls and Polish-smoked sausage.

●

Beef intestine casings are used for large-sized rolls, such as bologna and salami. Collagen casings come in a variety of sizes and lengths, according to what is being placed inside them. Synthetic casings can also be manufactured in numerous sizes.

Now, let's talk about what is used inside of some of these hot dogs that might alarm you. The next time you are in the market, check and see if the hot dog brand that you like contains "variety meats," which actually includes chicken livers, kidneys and hearts.

The U.S. Department of Agriculture requires that this information be disclosed on the ingredient label as "with variety meats" or "with meat by-products." This meat by product might also contain crushed bits of bone and cartilage among other things. I was surprised at first too.

Also, be sure to watch out for statements like "made with mechanically separated meats (MSM)." Mechanically separated meat is "a paste-like and batter-like meat product produced by forcing bones, with attached edible meat under high pressure through a sieve, or similar device, to separate the bone from the edible meat tissue," according to the U.S. Food Safety and Inspection Service (FSIS).

Although the FSIS maintains that MSM is safe to eat, only mechanically separated beef is no longer allowed in hot dogs and some other processed meats (as of 2004) because of fears of mad cow disease. Hot dogs can still contain no more than 20 percent mechanically separated pork and any amount of mechanically separated chicken or turkey. Only 20 percent? Yuck!

So if you're looking for the purest franks, pick those that are labeled "all beef," "all pork," or "all chicken, turkey, etc." Hot dogs labeled in this way must be made with meat from a single species and do not include byproducts. Even if they say it, I would still read the label anyway just to be on the safe side.

You should also know that turkey and chicken franks, for instance, can include turkey or chicken meat and turkey or chicken skin and fat in proportion to a turkey or chicken's carcass. With that in mind, ask yourself in a country that eats 20 billion hot dogs a year, with 9% being eaten at baseball games alone, are they even safe for you and your family to even eat?

You should know that eating lots of any processed meats, like hot dogs, has been linked to an increased risk of some cancers. Part of that risk is probably due to the additives used in the meats, namely sodium nitrite and MSG, or monosodium glutamate.

Sodium nitrite, (or sodium nitrate,) is used as a preservative, coloring and flavoring in hot dogs (and other processed meats), and studies have found it can lead to the formation of cancer-causing chemicals called nitrosamines. This is a cause for alarm.

MSG is a flavor enhancer used in hot dogs and many other processed foods and has been labeled as an "excitotoxin," which, are "a group of excitatory amino acids that can cause sensitive neurons in the brain to die." Though MSG has been labeled as a safe additive, some people's reactions to it should offer some kind of warning. Are you allergic to it? It is better to be on the safe side of any foods that you eat to know.

You should also know that a hot dog is just the tip of the iceberg of disturbing facts about foods that we eat. For instance, that collagen used in hot dogs is also the very same reason why gelatin, or Jello, actually gets to jiggle like that. It is filled with collagen, which as I said is derived from animal skin, often pigs. Then, this gelatin is also used as a thickening agent, which is then used in cereals, especially, frosted ones, some yogurts, candy and some types of sour cream.

Also, as you know, carbon monoxide is one of the most deadly gases on earth. So why is it in our food? The same stuff that comes from the exhaust pipe in your car is being used to packages ground beef and fish, such as tuna. Why? It keeps that meat from turning brown.

After all the air, which is why the meat turns brown, is taken out. Carbon monoxide is injected in. The best part is that this practice isn't widely used any more. That's because many people believe that this practice helps hide the fact that a lot of this food actually went bad.

The next time that you want to shove a whole handful of jelly beans or anything with a candy coating in your mouth, stop yourself! These shiny treats have been coated with a substance called shellac, which is found in the secretions of a female bug from Thailand called the female Kerria lacca. Sure they call it "confectioner's glaze" on the packaging, but now that you know what it is, what will you call it? Will you even still eat it?

Speaking of insects, the food industry has another way to use them in your favorite foods. They are good sources of color, especially the color red. Using boiled cochineal bugs, which are a type of beetle, the food industry extracts what is commonly called carmine. Carmine is a red food-coloring used in many foods.

The number one concern for you and your family is that this bug-based coloring can cause severe allergic reactions in some people, including potentially life-threatening anaphylactic reactions just like when people are allergic to peanuts or shellfish. Because of this, any food with this extract has to be clearly labeled. Carmine is often found in ice cream, Skittles candies, lemonade and grapefruit juice. Check the label to see if it is there.

As you know too much salt can contribute to high blood pressure and other health issues. Whoever said that I want more of it in my food? This extra salt is added through a process called plumping, where salt and other ingredients are injected into meats, like chicken, to enhance the flavor and increase the weight of it before it is sold. Yes, a lot of that weight could be salt water.

If you have to buy one of these prepackaged meats, check the label. If the label says "flavored with up to 10% of a solution" or "up to 15% chicken broth," avoid it. It may have five times the sodium of an ordinary piece of chicken. Any seasoning that you add could send your sodium or salt level through the roof.

I also love the beach. I just hate it when I get sand into my bathing suit and my hair. I just don't know how it got into my food. Silicon dioxide, which we call sand, does a great job of making sure things flow. So it is often in foods that need to pour easily. This sand can be as close as some soups and coffee creamers. Always check the label for sodium dioxide. It's extra salt.

It is also known that ammonia, which is a strong smelling chemical, is good for cleaning. It is used in glass cleaners. I just don't want it in my foods. Yet, there it is. Ammonia is also a gas that was once widely used to kill bacteria and germs on fatty beef trimmings. These trimmings have the most bacteria on it. The result is a pink slime that is used as filler in ground beef.

By now, we all have heard about this pink slime that comes from those little bits of meat that clings to fat. This fat is melted to remove it from the meat. They call this filler lean, finely textured beef. It is then treated with the ammonia and added to your ground beef. How much ground beef? About 10 billion pounds per year!

In the news, many fast food restaurants and supermarkets have been forced to report if their hamburgers have this pink slime. Some did and some didn't. Some markets reported that they would no longer carry it. Schools now have a choice of ordering beef without it, which is good news for all children.

Are you still with me? Good. Brace yourself. The next time that you are at the doctors and the doctor prescribes an antibiotic, take it as your doctor prescribed you to. It helps fight infections that could possibly harm you. But, when it comes to some livestock, like beef and chicken, the same antibiotics are being used by their producers to help these animals grow bigger, faster and make the producers even more money. It also might be harming you.

That's because antibiotics are only meant to fight germs. Abuse can lead to a growing problem of antibiotic resistance. Over time, the bacteria could then develop ways to get around the effectiveness of the antibiotics. Then, when we do need them, they might not work as effectively, which could lead to food borne illnesses. That's why I suggest grass fed livestock.

This is also why I have always made a point of telling people exactly what they are eating. This will allow them to change how they are eating, and then, feel better about the choices that they make in the foods that they are eating. It will also help them avoid the wrong foods.

Eating healthier is all about awareness. Awareness is what brings about change. At some point, we all will have to eat something that we know isn't really good for us. But, awareness also allows us to exercise moderation in what we eat. For instance, I still eat and love cookies. But, you should also know that because I know what is in some of them, like hydrogenated oils, which is bad for you, I don't always eat as much as I used to.

Since I want to maintain my weight loss, I only eat what is recommended as a serving. There is a reason why it they have recommended serving sizes, so that you won't overdo it. Sure there are times when you might want a little bit more, but that doesn't always mean you should. By the time that your mind realizes that you have had enough, you might have already overeaten.

Trust me, I don't really like to tell people exactly what to eat and when to eat, because everybody is different and it's up to you to make the proper choices in the foods that you eat. Again, this comes from listening to your body which will tell you when to eat, how much and when to stop. When was the last time that you did this?

You should always remember that what works for me, may not work for you. So in this book, I will suggest certain foods to add to what you already eat. What you add can make more of a difference than what you might take away. The healthier that the foods that you add are, the better that they will be for you in the end.

Never be afraid to experiment to find out which ones are right for you and what amounts. My concern is what is in these foods and what has to be done to get them to your table or make them more appealing to you. Contrary to popular belief not all processed foods are bad for you. It's the fat, sat and added sugar that signals a cause for alarm.

Then, you have some diet plans and the media making your question everything that you eat and not always in a good way. I recently heard of a woman, who got a call from her mother upset because a new diet said all wheat, and more importantly, bread is bad for you.

You should know that every new diet needs a villain and most diets attack the foods that we already eat as being responsible for our being overweight. If certain foods are so bad, how come people have been able to survive on them for so long? You know what; let's talk more about breads and other processed foods. You might want to get comfortable. We have only reached the beginning of this topic...

Processed Food: From The Farm To Your Table

If you have ever told yourself that you shouldn't eat processed food. I am afraid that you wouldn't end up eating anything at all. In people's minds, they have it set up that all processed foods are bad for you. Not all processed foods are bad for you. Some are, but I am sure nobody ever explained to you just why that is.

The more than you tell yourself what you can't have them, especially when it comes to some processed foods, like potato chips, is the more that you will want them. The bottom line is that people tend to want what they can't have. Then, the minute that you give in; you tend to feel like a failure. You are not. Not when you have been eating other processed foods all along.

Even when a person is trying to quit smoking, you just cannot quit cold turkey. If you do, you are setting yourself up for failure, if and when you make a mistake. That is why I suggest that nobody ever just ever flat out quits certain foods. If you are drawn to sweet or salty snacks, you should start by reducing your portions and try not to eat them so often.

Most of the problems with processed foods stem from what is in these foods that you do not see in the process to get them from the farm to your dinner table. With most of these foods, you are eating them out of habit, or because it is convenient, such as hot dogs. Yes, you are making a huge mistake, but it is one that we can actually learn from.

You see processed foods are any foods that have been altered from their natural state for either safety reasons or for convenience. To get food from its natural source to your local supermarket or grocery store, and then, to your dinner table, often this food has been canned, frozen, refrigerated, dehydrated or processed in a way that removes any bacteria or other harm for you.

So, virtually all food is processed. What I want to do right now, is help you distinguish between what is right for you and what isn't. That's because when we think about processed foods, we often think about canned meals, anything out a box or most snacks. The truth is that the number one kind of processed food that we use is milk. Milk is actually good for you in a lot of ways. It is loaded with calcium and vitamin D, which we need.

The reason why milk is considered processed is because it goes through a process called pasteurization, which heats the milk to kill any bacteria right away, and then, quickly cools it off. It is also homogenized; a process that I can tell you is used to keep the fat in the milk from separating. Because of this pasteurization, some people prefer raw milk, which can cause food-borne illnesses. With that in mind, not all processed foods are bad for you. They are not.

If you freeze seasonal fruits like strawberries, you help preserve the vitamins and make it possible to have them all year round. Fruit and vegetable juices are examples of healthy food processing. Many juices, like orange juice, are also fortified with essential nutrients like calcium and Omega-3 to make them better for you.

The problem is that there are a lot of processed foods that aren't as good. They are often filled with trans fats, unhealthy saturated fats, large amounts of sugar and salt. These are the things that we need to avoid or cut back on. Many of these are foods that we can eat, but, just not every day, and in moderation. Foods like:

- ✓ Canned foods with large amounts of fat or salt
- ✓ Breads and pastas made with refined white flour
- ✓ Pre-package cakes, cookies and candies
- ✓ Boxed meals that are high in fat or salt
- ✓ Packaged meals that are high in fat or salt
- ✓ Fish products that are high in sodium
- ✓ Sugary breakfast cereals
- ✓ Processed meats, like deli meat and hot dogs

Why? The truth is again certain processed meats will increase your risk of developing certain types of cancers, including colorectal cancer, according to some health officials. Processed meats, like hot dogs, bologna, sausage and other packaged lunch meats are frequently higher in calories, saturated fat and salt.

Before you buy your next box of cereal, another processed food, check the label and see how healthy it is for you or your family. You will know it is, if it is made with 100% whole grain and fortified, that means having additional nutrients added, like iron. Many of the most popular cereals are very low in fiber and have too much sugar. When in doubt, read the label very carefully.

If you have to continue to eat any of these products out of convenience, or because you love them, then you should always balance it out with fresher foods, like fruits and vegetables. Eating an apple though won't make up for eating a bunch of TV dinners, but eating whole grain bread will help balance things out when eating a sandwich made with processed lunch meat.

Add a garden salad, fresh vegetables, or some whole grain bread will make any meal healthier. I will argue for including low fat cheese to anyone's diet. It helps promote weight loss and helps maintain muscle mass.

If you don't like salads, you might eat more of it if you knew that lettuce contains antioxidants. You hear a lot about antioxidants, but now, let me finally clue you in about them. Antioxidants are widely used in dietary supplements and have been investigated for the prevention of diseases, such as cancer and coronary heart disease. This is good news for you.

If you don't like mushrooms on your pizza, what if I told you that mushrooms help fight cancer? Are you anemic and suffer from low iron in your blood? Eat more shellfish, beans and fortified cereals to raise your iron levels. Again, every little bit helps, so eat more of it.

Need more vitamin D in your diet? You should then look no further than eggs, tuna, milk and cereal. Facing a calcium deficiency, drink more low-fat milk and eat more low-fat Greek yogurt. You'll also burn more fat. Diabetic? Tea helps to naturally lower your blood sugar.

Fruits and vegetables again come in every color of the rainbow. Colorful fruits and deeply colored fruits like egg plants are low in calories, but are packed with vitamins and minerals and fiber. Greens are a good source of calcium, magnesium, iron, potassium, zinc, and vitamins A, C, E and K. All of which are essential vitamins that could make a big difference in your life.

Small vegetables, like corn, carrots, beets, sweet potatoes, yams and onions, will help reduce your cravings for sweets. Fruits, like berries, will fill you with vitamins, fiber and antioxidants. An apple can provide even more fiber. Oranges have the most vitamin C.

Adding more fruits and vegetables to your diet will also save you time and money on buying supplements, because that's all they should be. They should be doctor prescribed supplements to helps balance deficiencies that you already have in your body. For any other vitamin, they should always come from the foods that you already eat every day. If not, why not?

With most diet plans and weight loss plans on the market, many times these plans often ignore the nutrition value of their plans. They are only concerned with making false promises about how fast you can lose weight. Even then, it as if the only word that they know is protein and the most feared word in any diet is carbs. Carbs. Carbs. Carbs. Let's talk about them right now...

The Truth About Carbs Is Not What You Think!

Every diet plan and weight loss on the planet is screaming about carbs, carbs, and more carbs! Enough already! Did you know that your body actually prefers carbs as its number one energy source?

With everything that is being said about carbs, it is often hard to tell which one is right and which one is wrong for you. Well, the answer is as close as the next sandwich that you make and the flour that your bread is made of.

When you make one sandwich with white bread, is it better for you than one made with whole grains? When you are at Wendy's should you order the fries or the chili? What about a side salad? Which one has the carbs? The truth is that they all have them.

The salad, chili and whole grain bread are just excellent source of good carbs because they contain whole grains and vegetables. Right now, we just have to learn how to separate the good from the bad and remember that it's the number of and quality of the calories, not the carbs, which make certain foods bad.

When you choose good carbs for your diet, you will find that these carbs tend to absorb slowly into your system, which helps your body avoid spikes in your blood sugar. If no one ever told you that spikes in blood sugar is regulated by your body. This is important to your weight loss, and more importantly, your ability to maintain it.

When there is a spike in blood sugar, your pancreas produces insulin and glucagon. This helps remove the excess blood sugar from the body, but it doesn't always remove the right amount. When your body sugar begins to get low, you tend to begin to crave some of the most sugary snacks available, snacks that may also contain a lot of fat and not enough fiber, which is bad for you.

Good carbs also contain fiber. If you are like most people, you probably are confused about fiber. Don't be ashamed. Most people are. You are not alone. The trick is that you don't have to know everything about how fiber works to benefit from what it can do.

Fiber is a type of carbohydrate, or carb, that the body can't digest. A good source of this is whole fruits and vegetables, whole grain breads and some whole grain breakfast cereals and all types of beans.

Contrary to popular belief, fiber is actually very good for you. It is fiber that helps you feel fuller longer. Fiber works best when teamed up with fluids, like water. Water actually helps expand your stomach causing your stomach to send that signal to your brain that you are full, enabling you to stop eating.

The excess water, then, helps to carry away the excess byproducts and it also helps burn up the excess fat. That is why you should always include high fiber, such as fruits and vegetables, in every meal or snack.

Fiber also slows down the absorption of other nutrients eaten at the same meal, including other carbohydrates. This slowing may help prevent those awful peaks and valleys in your blood sugar levels, reducing your risk for developing type 2 diabetes dramatically.

Certain types of fiber, especially the ones found in oats, beans, and some fruits can also help lower your blood cholesterol. This is essential for your heart health.

That's because it lowers your risk of having a heart attack, and even, your risk of having a stroke.

The problem is that you probably aren't eating anything that is already high in fiber. We are a society that lives off of white flour and white rice. Your bagel is made of it in the morning. The sandwich you ate at lunch had it and so does the white rice that you had for dinner.

The whiter the foods that we eat, especially bread, the lower the fiber. This is where bad carbs come in. We can also fight the health risks involved by limiting these bad carbs from our diets altogether.

That's because as I mentioned before the process used to make these items, often strip these foods of their most beneficial fibers. So contrary to what many diets will make you believe, not all carbs are bad for you.

The best way to get more fiber, and well, the only way to get it is by eating organic foods, such as anything that is grown like fruits and vegetables. Plants, like fruits and vegetables, are quality carbohydrates that are loaded with fiber. This again is fiber that your body needs and should get on a regular basis.

Would you eat more fiber in your diet if I told you that the chance of developing colon cancer is actually 1 in every 20 women? Fiber actually helps to promote colon health, not just weight control, reducing your chances of colon cancer. An apple a day can keep the doctor away.

That's why good carbs can only come from a plant and are not made in a plant. According to the Harvard University School of Public Health, there are five ways to add more fiber to your diet...

1. Eat whole fruits, instead of just drinking the juice. Whole apples and whole oranges are packed with a lot more fiber and a lot fewer calories than their juices.

2. The reason why we call it "breakfast" is because the last time most people ate was dinner, so you are essentially breaking your fasting or not eating. Break the fast with some fruit. Get off to a great start by adding fruit, like berries or melon, to your breakfast every day. It could easily be added to your hot oatmeal or cold cereal for a more nutritious and delicious meal.

3. Always check the label for fiber-filled whole grains for any foods that claim to have it. Choose foods that list whole grains (like whole wheat or oats) as the first ingredient. Bread, cereal, crackers and other grain foods should have at least 3 grams of fiber per serving.

4. Eat more beans. It's easy to forget about beans, but they are a great tasting, cheap source of fiber, good carbs, protein and other important nutrients.

5. Try a new dish. Test out international recipes that use whole grains, like tabouli, whole wheat pasta, or beans. The internet is filled with delicious recipes for them and so many other fiber loaded recipes.

As you experiment, try mixing whole grains to your regular ingredients, like adding a little whole grain pasta to the regular pasta into your spaghetti dinner and see if you can taste the difference. You won't.

You might be surprised that what is good for you will also taste good to you. Best of all, it is not depriving you of anything. If it is actually helping you, I say do it.

The goal is to only add good carbs via whole grains, fruits and vegetables to your diet. You have to make sure that you are getting the whole grains that you need, even when you are experimenting with a variety of them to find out what you like.

Labels that say things like stone, ground, multigrain or, even, 100 percent whole wheat can also be deceptive. The only way to know for sure is to look for the whole grain stamp that you will find on some foods, like cereal.

Bad carbs won't just go away though. Again, you should know that there will come a point where you have to eat foods that may not always be healthy for you and loaded with bad carbs. You can eat them or you can go hungry. That's the point where you have to exercise portion control and moderation.

Any other time, if we put real gas in our cars and feed our pet real food, why don't we do the same for ourselves? Some people actually feed their pets better than they feed themselves. Why?

Why should we continue to feed ourselves things that we know are bad for us or eat foods that have things in them that we can't even pronounce? We can't be good to ourselves, if we are not doing the things that are good for us, like eating healthier.

With this in mind, I think it's about time that I show you the ugly truth about these other carbs, these so called "bad carbs" that some diet plans harp on, but they never tell you exactly why or where to find them. Remember when I said that good carbs come from a plant, not made in a plant. Let me explain why bad carbs are not good for you and just where they really do come from...

Bad Carbs Are Made, Not Grown

The answer is simple. Good carbs are anything that comes from a plant that serves as food. It should be a good source of fiber, vitamins, and minerals.

The problem with bad carbs is that sometimes, they play a good game of hide and seek in your food that you will never be able to win at. Okay, sometimes you can, but only if you know what you are looking for.

Bad carbs are really just sugars, more specifically added sugars and those refined white grains. It doesn't help that you are probably already eating more sugar than ever before. It is the new drug and we simply have to have it and we will get it one way or another.

According to the American Heart Association, Americans eat about 22 teaspoons of sugar a day! That is about a half a cup of sugar day. If you weigh less than 160 pounds, you will end up consuming more than your body weight in sugar every year.

The truth is the average woman, according the American Heart Association should only eat about six. With eight teaspoons of sugar in just a 12 ounce can of soda, this will already put you over your daily limit for sugar intake, making this another reason why many people are losing in their battle to cut back on sweets.

It doesn't help that the government doesn't require labels to show you the difference between naturally occurring sugars and added ones. This would help in your attempt to cut back on that food or beverage. How can you practice moderation when you don't know when enough is enough? The key is to learn where to look for this extra sugar in some of your favorite foods.

When you read a label, check for things like cane and maple syrups, honey or molasses, brown rice syrup, cane juice, fruit juice concentrate, malt dextrin, dextrose, fructose or glucose. They are all hidden sources of sugar, when the USDA recommends that we get no more than 6% to 10% of our total calories from added sugar. That might be only 200 calories.

Another big problem is that sugar simply makes everything taste better. Sugar is a quick supply of energy in the form of glucose. This can be a good thing if you are competing in a race or a sports event. But, it's not a good idea if you are just sitting around on the couch and doing absolutely nothing.

Otherwise, the best sugars for you should come from fructose, which can be found naturally in fruit and lactose, which is found in milk. Lactose is the sugar that some people can't break down in their body, which leads to lactose intolerance. For those who are lactose intolerant, you can still get the calcium that you need through items such as calcium-fortified orange juice.

With a lot of this added sugars, most of it is added during the processing of these foods, like high fructose corn syrup used in soda and many baked goods, like cakes and cookies. This game of hide and seek gets even worst when people in their attempts to lose weight begin to eat more fat-free and low-fat foods also.

According to United States Department of Agriculture, which regulates food safety in this country, what most people don't know is that added sugar is often substituted for fat in many low fat foods. They had to do something to make it taste better for you. So, they added sugar. How much sugar? Too much of it.

There is an alternative. For instance, if you need to add something sweet to your food or drink, like tea, I would suggest raw sugar or honey. Honey has begun to show great promise in helping to reduce weight gain when substituted for sugar.

Honey is a nutritious fat releasing alternative that also boasts antibacterial, antiviral, and antifungal properties. It will actually help improve the control of your blood sugar. Try it with some green tea.

When you are feeling a craving coming on for something sweet, again look no further than a piece of fruit to curb your sugar craving. Also, make sure that you aren't skipping meals. That is the reason why your body may be producing such intense food cravings.

This condition is caused by your body's lowered blood sugar levels because you haven't eaten. The lower your blood sugar levels, the more cravings that you will have. This is why hungry chicks should never go hungry.

After your weight loss, you will see that the lighter your body has become, the less energy that you need to do basic things. This will give you the energy to do more of the things that you like to do and the more active that you will become, the more fat burning that you will also be able to do. This will finally give you that flatter belly that you have been dreaming about for years.

Speaking of fats, it's time that we talk about that too. Another word of caution, don't believe everything that some plans have told you about fats. Eating fat doesn't always cause fat. If it did, why are lean cuts of pork actually good for you...

Don't Believe The Hype About Fats!

Ask the average person what do they know about saturated fat and they probably will tell you that it causes heart disease. Then, ask that same person what do they know about cholesterol and they will tell you that it is bad for you. For years, I would have said the very same thing and I was trained in the culinary arts.

As a chef, I have always wondered why if you didn't need fat in your diet, why would they continue to sell low fat foods? Why not remove all of the fat? For the past twenty years, we all have been encouraged to believe that saturated fats and cholesterol, both found in animal fats, are the main causes of chronic degenerative diseases. In some ways, this is true. But, what happens when we don't get any at all?

Contrary to popular belief, we still need that saturated fat. It actually provides strength and rigidity to our cells. It helps enhance our immune system. It helps incorporate calcium into our bones. Some fat also helps protect us from bacteria in our digestive system.

Cholesterol actually provides additional much needed strength to our cells. It helps convert Vitamin D, which is essential to strong bones and teeth. It provides muscle tone and helps our immune system function properly. Cholesterol also acts as an antioxidant by protecting our bodies from cellular damage that causes cancer and heart disease. How can something like that be bad?

The truth is that there is a good and a bad side to everything, including saturated fats and cholesterol, the same way that there is for carbohydrates. The danger in both of these naturally occurring things is when they have been damaged by heat, oxygen or unnatural farming practices. This is the problem, not the fat itself.

This damaged fat and cholesterol is actually what causes damage to arteries and actually promotes the build up of a plaque that is then used to heal the injured areas of the heart. This build up causes problems with your blood circulation and is the beginning stages of heart disease and other chronic illnesses.

The problem for all of us is that we eat many of these products every day and we don't even realize it. One of the main sources of this damaged fat and cholesterol is pasteurized dairy products, which includes cheese and ice cream made from these pasteurized dairy products.

Pasteurization, which I mentioned before, is the process of heating milk, and then, immediately cooling it to slow down the growth of microbiotic bacteria, which damages the fat and cholesterol in these products and everything made from them. Again, everything has the potential to be harmful if you eat or drink too much of it. That is why even though dairy is good for you, you should still exercise moderation and limit your servings.

Another source is any meat that has been cooked at extremely high temperatures, especially those that have been deep fried. To do this, many times, you are required to use a vegetable oil or some other hydrogenated oil. These oils have been chemically changed to stabilize them and ensure their shelf life.

So, with that in mind, you probably are wondering how we can still get this healthy fat and cholesterol, if these certain types of foods should be limited. The answer is there are still many other healthy sources, including nuts, cold-water fish, organic eggs, organic chicken, grass fed beef, virgin coconut oil and olive oil.

The difference in organic and non-organic food is what makes all of the difference. For instance, let's look at the difference between organic and non-organic eggs. Our body functions best when we have a healthy balance of omega-6 and omega-3 fatty acids.

The right amount of omega-3 triggers fat burning enzymes. Having too much or too little can lead to many health issues down the road, including high blood pressure, and yes, weight gain.

With organic eggs, when a hen is allowed to eat green plants and naturally occurring foods, then, the eggs produced have the best balance of these fatty acids. This balance is 1:1 in omega-6 and omega-3 fatty acids. This is good for us. When it comes to commercially raised eggs, this ratio is often a high as 15:1 or 20:1. That is 15 or 20 times the recommended amount.

Omega-3 and omega-6 fatty acids can also be found in fish, such as salmon, herring, mackerel and sardines. It is also readily available in soybeans, corn and walnuts. These fats have been proven to help release body fat, especially that dreaded belly fat.

That's because these types of fats have a higher resting metabolic rate, which is the calories used just to live and are the easiest to burn off when you are trying to lose weight. It is also easier to feel full when eating these types of fats. That's why, again, the next time you are hungry for a snack, reach for a hand full of almonds, hazelnuts or pecans. They are also known to help improve your mood as well. All you need is a hand full.

When we cook, since we still need this healthy fat in our diet, try virgin coconut oil and red palm oil. They are the best oils to cook with because they contain a large percentage of saturated fats that remain stable and undamaged with heat. If you need to cook with more oil, try canola oil, peanut oil or olive oil.

All other vegetable oils are damaged easily with heat exposure and the number one way that we use these oils is at high temperatures to fry foods. Also, try cold-pressed olive oil, which is best eaten raw. This is the same oil provided to you with any bread at an Italian restaurant. It is a delicious and nutritious source of fat.

Speaking of fats, let's dispel another myth right now. All fat doesn't make you fat. You actually have to eat some fat to fight being fat. So if you are looking to improve your overall health and still lose weight, a diet rich in these good fats can help.

It is only when you eat too much of the wrong fat, as in those found in highly processed meat and some cookies, that's when these fats become bad for you. Again, always exercise moderation.

Going back to our childhood, one of the best snacks we ever had was that peanut butter and jelly sandwich is a smart choice. Eat one now as an adult. Peanut butter is a monounsaturated fat, or MUFA, which is good for you and fights belly fat too. Eat some of it.

What's more, these kinds of fats, actually helps you to feel fuller—they have 9 calories per gram compared to 4 for protein or carbs. So a small nibble of something delicious, like a handful of nuts, or that peanut butter on whole wheat crackers, can help you feel full for hours.

Remember, our ultimate goal is to look better, eat better, feel better and have more energy. When you eat the right balance of fatty acids it will show not just in your waist, but also you hair, nails and skin as well. That's why you will look better. That is also why it is always best to focus on foods that rich in omega-3 fatty acids, which can help your entire body. Foods like:

✓ Halibut	✓ Salmon
✓ Herring	✓ Sardines
✓ Mackerel	✓ Trout
✓ Oysters	✓ Tuna (fresh)

The best part is that in this day and age, you don't have to look far to find anything fortified with omega-3. Fortified foods are defined as any food that can provide these health benefits beyond just basic nutrition.

These days, supermarkets are filled to the brim with everything from fortified juice to eggs produced by chickens fed omega-3s in their grain. You will most likely find the following foods fortified with omega-3 fatty acids, if you look:

✓ Eggs	✓ Juice
✓ Margarine	✓ Soy milk
✓ Milk	✓ Greek yogurt

Some breads and pasta are also just some of the foods most commonly enriched with omega-3. You'll also find them in whole foods like seeds and nuts. When shopping, look for omega-3 in wheat breads, cereals, crunchy oats, flour, whole wheat pasta, peanut butter, oatmeal, pumpkin seeds, flour tortillas and walnuts.

Vegetables, especially green leafy ones, are rich in ALA, another form of omega-3 fatty acids. Although ALA isn't as powerful as the other omega-3 fatty acids, DHA and EPA, these vegetables also offer a host of benefits, from fiber to antioxidants, in addition to the omega-3. This includes Brussels sprouts, spinach or watercress lettuce that you can use in your salad.

Speaking of eating salads, there is another dieting mistake that millions of people make when trying to lose weight. While a big salad might seem healthy, when you load it down with bacon bits, croutons and cheese crumbs, it becomes no different than a big pasta meal.

Why? Think about how much salad dressing that you put on a salad. You should only put enough to coat your salad. If there is dressing at the bottom after you eat, you have eaten way too much. Remember that most salad dressings are made with fat and oils. You can save up to 500 calories, just by limiting your salad to one topping, such as roasted onions or peppers and using only half of your usual low fat dressing.

Whatever you do, try to reduce or eliminate as much saturated fats, such as the fatty cuts of red meats and whole milk as possible. Trust me; one or two percent milk eventually won't taste any different in your morning coffee or cereal. It might even taste better to you.

Also, limit or reduce the amount of trans fats in your food, which include vegetable shortening, margarine, cookies, candies, fried foods and some baked food if the labels say hydrogenated oils. These are the bad fats. That's because like pasteurized milk, these healthy fats and cholesterol has been damaged by heat.

Also, learn what fat is in most foods just by their title on a menu or in a cookbook. To avoid foods with unhealthy saturated fat and cholesterol, steer clear of any foods that says au gratin, basted, battered, breaded, buttery, buttered, in butter sauce, casserole, cheesy, creamed, creamy, crispy, deep-fried, escalloped, fried, gooey, gravy, hash, hollandaise, marinated (in oil), pan-fried, parmesan, pot pie, prime, refried, sauce (cream sauce, cheese sauce), sautéed, tempura and white sauce. If you can't cut them out eventually altogether, use moderation and limit what you eat to the recommended serving size

Again, you don't have to give up everything that you love. But, just make a few smart changes or substitutions. For example, the next time that you are in the market, pick up some toasted sesame oil or fruit juice to cook with or macadamia nut oil to make something as simple as pancakes with. Love butter, try walnut oil. You will love it just as much.

Now that we have gotten that out the way, let's talk about the new secret weapon in the battle of the bulge...protein. Sure you have heard a lot about it. Let's talk briefly about how to make it work for you...

Protein – The Secret Weapon In Weight Loss

Most people are afraid of protein. Why? They think that the only way that they can get this protein is from greasy fried chicken or a steak that takes the body 72 hours to digest. The truth is that good protein is as close as your next helping of skinless white meat chicken, turkey, seafood, low fat dairy, pork tenderloins, beans and nuts, like pistachios, lean beef and eggs. That is why eggs are always a good way to start off your day.

These high protein foods often take longer to digest and metabolize, which encourages our bodies to burn more calories. Maybe that is why protein has become the new secret weapon in weight loss. That's because protein is more satisfying to your body than any carb on the planet. It is not only good for you, but good to you.

Protein is what gives us the energy to get up and go. Protein is what strengthens your muscles and keeps the amount of fat in your body in check. The problem is that almost one-third of all women don't get enough protein, even if they aren't trying to lose weight. This is another big mistake for all women.

Protein, in food, is actually broken down into the 20 amino acids that are the body's building blocks for growth and energy. It is also essential for maintaining healthy cells, tissue and every organ in your body.

The best part of all of this is that you don't always need to have a lot of it to reap its benefits. Focus on fresh fish, turkey, chicken and eggs, which are excellent sources of protein. Then, eat them. That's it. Next, still think dairy will hurt your diet? It won't, let me tell you why...

The Reason Why You Should Eat More Dairy...

Given what we now know about fatty acids, and even, with the dangers of pasteurization, let's put another myth to rest right now about how eating dairy products, like cheese, will hurt your weight loss efforts and your health. If you want to believe that still, you're wrong.

Research has proven that nothing could be further from the truth. It is only when you aren't getting enough calcium and you have a calcium deficiency will you lose your control over your appetite, causing you to gain more weight. The solution, eat more low fat dairy.

Eating low fat dairy is very effective in accelerating fat loss and helps eliminate some of the risk brought on by pasteurization. That's because you need the calcium, which once in your body helps to regulate your fat storage. A high calcium diet will turn more of those calories into heat than body fat, which leads to the loss of your belly fat, giving you a flatter stomach.

With a balanced diet and lower caloric intake, by adding just three servings a day, you too will see acceleration in your fat loss and weight loss. These servings could come as easily as a glass of low fat milk for breakfast with your morning eggs, a snack of low fat cheese, and a cup of low fat Greek yogurt, which I mentioned, is actually better for you, as a snack.

Remember that low fat yogurt contains something called probiotics. Probiotics are friendly bacteria that research suggests may actually help reduce the amount of fat that your body absorbs. Try it. You will see the results.

More importantly, low fat cheese and yogurt could provide more calcium. This calcium is essential for strong bones and teeth. But whoever said that you had to eat actual dairy products to get more calcium in your diet to reap the benefits.

If you are lactose intolerant, this means your body can't digest lactose, the natural sugar in milk; I would suggest you trying fat free milk or one or two percent milk or fortified orange juice.

Another excellent source of calcium is spinach and cereals fortified with calcium. Almond butter is a good source, and even, figs. Don't forget cabbage, celery and broccoli. Now, eat more of it.

Just remember to exercise moderation and always make sure that any dairy you consume is low fat. I took whole milk off my shopping list years ago. Why? It is actually more fattening than you think. There is another hidden danger that I will talk about later.

For now, just know that low fat dairy products not only reduce the risks, but you can still reap the rewards of that dairy product, in terms of calcium and vitamin D. But, again, exercise moderation. You shouldn't have more than three servings per day. That's all you need.

Now that we have talked about some of the things that we should have, let me talk about something else that you should only have in small doses. Remember, a lot of the weight that you now have is water weight because of one culprit--salt. It's time that we finally talk about it...

Salt...It's Not Just A Movie With Angelina Jolie.

The same way that sugar plays a game of hide and seek in your food, you should also know that salt is often more clever. Once used to preserve just about everything, salt is often one of your worst enemies when it comes to trying to lose weight and keep it off.

That's because you might be consuming high levels of hidden salts in your foods, like some breads, canned soups, pasta sauces, margarine, frozen dinners, instant mashed potatoes, and even, ketchup. Yes, ketchup!

When we add salt to our food when we cook, or while we are eating, we do it because we think it will improve the taste. When processed food is made, extra salt has already added to improve the taste and help keep the food fresher longer. Even then, salt is already naturally found in most foods. When you add table salt, it only increases the amount of the salt in it. This is what makes things bad for you.

With more than one-third of American adults considered obese, this is about to become the most important conversation that we will ever have. That's because more than likely, you are already consuming too much salt. When you read your label, the first time that you see the word "sodium" in your ingredients, you have found the first source of salt in it. The closer to the beginning of the ingredients it is, the more salt there is.

So why is salt so important to your weight loss efforts? You should know that salt itself does not cause your body to gain or lose fat. In fact, salt doesn't have any calories. But, when you continuously consume high amounts of salt, this will result in you gaining weight because it causes your body to retain the empty calories from sodas or juice that you used to quench your thirst. This is where most of your bad calories are.

You see our bodies rely on salt for its electrolytes. These electrolytes carry the necessary electrical impulses that control certain signals that we need for our bodies to function properly, making it very important to maintain this balance. When our electrolytes are high, this causes our body to become thirsty. We should then be drinking enough water to correct this imbalance.

Movie theaters, bars and restaurants know this. This is why bars always provide you with free chips, pretzels and peanuts, all salty foods, so that you will buy more drinks. The more you eat it, the thirstier you will become, and the more money that they will make.

When we do drink enough water, your body responds via your kidneys by controlling how much water you will retain to improve the amount of electrolytes in your body. The amount of water that you retain, in turn, will actually also helps to lower your blood pressure.

When the amount of salt is elevated in your body and we don't drink enough water, the water that we did consume will not just stay in our system or our bloodstream; it tends to move to our skin giving us that bloated look. When we reduce our salt intake, the body works in reverse by removing as much water from our system as possible, which is better for us. So the message here is to eat less salty foods and if you do eat a lot of salty food, drink enough water.

Before I go any further, let me tell you how our bodies even got to this point. The truth is that high levels of salt in our diets usually come from foods filled with empty calories, low in fiber, and basically, most processed foods like those found in fast foods restaurants and some on your favorite supermarket shelves. We have been eating so much of it that we don't even realize that we were doing it. This has never been a good thing.

When you reduce your salt intake, this can only help you to lose weight, because without the extra salt in your body, your body no longer feels a need to hold on to the extra water in your body. It is then free to expel it and the weight in your body that goes along with it.

The minute that you start eating salty food, the weight will come right back. Then what? In order for you to reach your ideal weight, this water weight might be the only weight that you have to lose. So continue to cut back on the salt, whenever and however possible.

The one thing that you should know is that it is often very hard to do anything about the salt that is already in most restaurant foods. But even, if you do eat out a lot, you still can do something about the other sources of sodium or salt in your diet, like not adding extra salt to your food at the table. You will see immediate results.

When you do eat out or at home, you definitely should not add extra salt to the food already loaded with it. If you are used to adding a lot of salt when you cook, try to go spicy or find another salt substitute, like curry, Mrs. Dash or pepper.

If you find yourself adding more salt to your food remember that this is purely out of habit. The more that you eat of it, the more you want it. Once you stop adding salt, you will discover the other flavors in your food that you will enjoy and that you have really been missing all along. It has been there, but you drowned it out by adding so much salt.

Also, remember that you will never be able to count up all of the salt that you eat all day. So my recommendation for you is to pretend that you are already in a high risk group for high blood pressure and lower the amount of salt that you eat. Again, first you have to avoid food containing large amounts of salt. You'll know when you see words like: in broth, in cocktail sauce, in tomato base or pickled.

At your table, remove the salt shakers and you remove the temptation. I can't remember the last time that I actually bought salt. Whenever possible, even in your shopping, opt for fresh or frozen, instead of canned. If you can't, choose low salt or low sodium products.

When it comes to seasoning your food, try a little sugar instead. You can even add a tablespoon of sugar when you cook to your corn or peas. This move often curbs my cravings for sugar, and ultimately, this helps to satisfy my sweet tooth as well. Try it and see what it can do for yours.

One thing that you can do right away is to stop drinking whole milk, you should know it actually contains more salt than you could imagine. Try 1%, 2% or skim. Speaking of drinking, let's talk about water. You probably spent more time showering in it than drinking it. Let me show you how to use it to change your life...

Water! Water! Water! It Is Everywhere, But How Much Do You Actually Take The Time To Drink...

How much water do you actually drink during the day? A cup disguised as your morning coffee? Did you drink a soda at lunch? Did you have a glass of juice at dinner? Soda, juice, and coffee, sure it's a liquid but, it's not the one thing that your body really needs—actual water.

The truth is the only time that most of us see actual water is on the table before a meal at a restaurant. Often, we don't even drink that. We just don't drink enough water, which our body needs for good health, even though we know that it is good for us.

It is estimated that 75% of all Americans are dehydrated. That's over 200 million people, not just celebrities. The problem is most people often mistake thirst for hunger and they will eat something faster than they will drink something. This is the biggest dieting mistake that most people make every single day, even if you are trying to lose weight or not.

Water actually regulates your body temperature, removes waste, transports nutrients to cells, cushions joints and protects your vital organs, restores the fluids lost by perspiration and other natural body functions. Water helps flush out unnecessary waste products, salts and toxins from our bodies. Without water, your body doesn't stand a chance to function properly.

If you intend to lose weight, you should already be drinking enough water every day anyway. How much? You should know that it isn't the eight to ten glasses that everybody thinks. This amount actually varies from person to person based on your actual weight. To find out how much, take your actual body weight and divide it by two. The result is your water number or how much water in ounces, preferably filtered water, which removes a lot of toxins that are found in local tap water, which you need to drink in order to maintain good health.

For example, let's say that you weigh 120 pounds. Divide that by two and you will get 60 ounces. Those 60 ounces, divided by 8 which is the number of ounces in a cup, is about the 7 and a half cups of water or more that you need to drink, especially if you have a very active lifestyle, or if you sweat a lot.

You should know that drinking water is also the best way to fight back against bloating and unnecessary water weight gain, which is caused by your body attempting to hold on to every bit of water that it can get. Bloating, as I mentioned before, is already a sure sign that you simply aren't drinking enough water and you have too much salt in your body. That's because salt also leeches water from the body, which only leads to further dehydration, bloating and water weight gain.

This is also important news for women, who suffer from monthly menstrual bloating. This kind of bloating usually starts a week before your cycle starts when you may be craving chocolate, chips and other sugary or salty snacks. This is the time that you should avoid them the most and drink more water. It will help with cramps too.

In any situation, try to think of water as your most important food group. The key is to take the time to drink enough of it. The problem is that many people will reach for a soda to quench their thirst or as a pick me up. That caffeine often will only make you feel even thirstier. Did you know that by replacing just one of these sodas a day with water, you can significantly reduce your caloric intake on any given day? Imagine the results of you replacing just two sodas a day with two glasses of ice cold water.

You should also know that thirst is the number one cause of afternoon fatigue, which causes your body to work harder to pump blood through your system, causing severe headaches. So, use whatever excuse that you can to drink more water. Carry a bottle with you that you can quickly refill to make sure that you are drinking enough water, and then, do it. Drink more water.

You should also drink water like this all year long. Some people think you only need to drink water like this when the weather is hot. You need to drink water like this even in the winter. The number one sign of dehydration in winter is dry skin, fatigue and cracked lips.

Also, don't be afraid to revisit your water number as you lose weight. The less that you weigh, the less water that you will need. In any situation, also make sure that you do not to overdo it, drinking too much water can cause other problems. That's because it lowers the body's natural sodium levels that the body needs, which can shut down a person's kidneys and prove to be fatal.

People instead should stick to drinking less than four glasses of water an hour. That's all that a person's kidneys can actually handle. If you stop and think about how little water that we do drink, it shouldn't be a surprise how easily it is for skip one of the most important meals of the day too--breakfast...

The Most Important Meal Of The Day…Breakfast

What if I told you that you could lose more weight simply by eating breakfast? In our busy society, who has the time? We spend more time on our daily commute than we do enjoying breakfast. We should be eating early, and then, eat often to keep your metabolism fire going.

To combat our guilt about this, we often tell ourselves that we are not hungry or that we just don't have time. The problem with that logic is that, in the end, we will pay for this too eventually. If we are lucky some mornings, we may get a leftover donut in our job's break room. At lunch time, we are starving.

Breakfast, as you already know, is the breaking of your fasting period of a night of not eating. The last meal that you probably had was dinner. If you are not hungry in the morning, the truth is you probably overdid it at dinner. If you are starving, you didn't eat enough.

When it comes to breakfast, whoever said that it has to be elaborate. Keep it simple. The only rule that you should follow is that you should eat within two hours of waking up. This lets your body know that you aren't starving and helps fight that starvation mode that I mentioned before. Remember food is information. It tells the body what to do, when and how to do it.

Eating breakfast will allow you to eat smaller meals throughout the day. When you don't eat breakfast, you tend to overcompensate for that by eating more at lunch or dinner. Your body has already begun to see this pattern causing it to store more calories than it needs to prevent you from going hungry for too long. So you see that you really can't afford to skip breakfast.

That's why breakfast is considered the most important meal of the day. You need to remember that before you attempt to skip it. Again, it doesn't have to fancy, just good for you. Even then, remember to keep it simple. Here are just a few breakfast ideas that might help:

Monday: Whole grain toast, apple butter, a glass of milk and piece of fruit.

Tuesday: Apple slices with peanut butter and milk

Wednesday: A mini bagel with reduced fat cream cheese and a small glass of juice.

Thursday: Low fat Greek yogurt with fresh strawberries and a glass of juice, and maybe, some toast

Friday: A bowl of apple cinnamon oatmeal or strawberries and cream, a piece of fruit and skim milk

Saturday: A breakfast rollup of scramble eggs on a flour tortilla with green peppers and onions and a glass of orange juice.

Sunday: Two pancakes or waffles, a glass of milk, eggs and two pieces of turkey bacon

It seems overwhelming at first, but it is doable. Now that we have talked about the most important meal, let's talk about something more complicated…eating out. In our busy lives, eating out is more convenient than ever. Can it still be healthy, let's find out together…

Can You Still Eat Out? Here's How...

Did you know that the color red often triggers hunger? This color is also often used in most fast food restaurant signs. KFC, Hardees, McDonald's, Pizza Hut, Burger King and convenience stores have what color on their roofs, buildings and signs? It's red. You may not have been hungry until you looked at the sign or the roof.

When you see red, suddenly, you have the urge for a shake, fries and a burger. That is not a coincidence. Despite a need to eat better, sometimes, eating away from home becomes unavoidable. Often a fast food or other dining outlet is often a quick fix to any hunger problem. You can make it work, but do you know how?

Since most restaurants only care about your taste buds and not about your waistline, it is often up to you to make eating out work. Given how quickly serving sizes have ballooned, you can easily face your biggest setback from just one night of eating if you aren't careful.

One of the biggest weapons that you have in your battle to eat healthier is their internet menus. Most restaurants post their menus online so that you know what you can eat before you get there. So know before you go what is on the menu and you won't be tempted to overdo it.

I also try to order first so that I am not tempted after whoever I am eating with orders a steak and a big baked potato with sour cream to do the same. Also, when I eat out, I am not afraid to substitute the white rice for another order of broccoli or the corn, which is a vegetable, but, it is still considered a starch.

I also try not to get seduced by the menu. The high priced items always come with a mouthwatering picture. The ribs and the steak will look so good. The dessert menu alone looks so good that you want to eat the picture. With me, I have already made up my mind before I left home and I stick to what I know and what I can eat responsibly and what is healthier.

The key here is also portion control. The 12 ounce steak might only be few bucks more. Who doesn't love a good deal? But, unless I am planning to make two meals out of it, dinner now and lunch tomorrow, I will pass on the bigger steak. Who needs the extra calories?

If it will become lunch tomorrow, I put it in another container, and then, freeze it. It will thaw out on my desk, and then, I can just pop it in the microwave when I am ready to eat. This keeps me from having it as a midnight snack and ruining my efforts to lose weight.

When eating out, remember the appetizer is just as important as the meal. I would suggest having the soup or the salad. You salad should be filled with as many leafy green vegetables as possible with a light dressing. If it is not on the menu, ask for it. They should have it.

If you order the soup, pick a broth based soup, like chicken noodle to help fill you up quicker. I am also not afraid of making a meal out of just appetizers. That's right appetizers, like those sliders or a soup and salad.

Unless you know that the bread basket is whole wheat, skip it. Instead, try a shrimp cocktail. You can still have the bread, but always try to hold it off until the end or eat it alongside your meal. If you know that the main course, or your dessert, is going to be large, offer to split it with your dinner companion. Or plan on only eating half. You are no longer a member of the clean plate club.

If you are really concerned about what you are about to eat, don't be afraid to order off the kid's menu. If it good enough for a child, why can't it be good enough for you? Order it without embarrassment. The best chicken that I have ever eaten came off the kid's menu of a Wolfgang Puck restaurant in Florida. It came complete with steamed baby carrots. It couldn't have been any healthier than it already was.

Your serving of meat, fish, chicken or beef, should never be any bigger than a deck of playing cards. And that bread that you love, make sure that your portion isn't bigger than a CD case. If you splurge and order dessert, if you can, take a walk to burn some of those calories off.

If it is a party that you are attending, my suggestion is that you eat before you go. That way you don't overdo it, especially if dinner isn't being served right away. You might be starving by the time that dinner is served.

So, you can eat out, as you can see, but make it on your terms. Eat instinctively or intuitively. Eat what you want, when you are hungry and as much as you should to fulfill your hunger. Also, when in doubt, substitute something out. You don't have to eat what is offered.

Don't be afraid to ask for something else and have it your way. Your speaking up now will help you do something more important in our next step. It is something millions of people are afraid to do…

The Most Important Step Now...Getting Help

The dirtiest words in the English language these days seem to be fat and diet. Suddenly, because of your need to lose a few pounds, you often feel ashamed or embarrassed. The truth is that you should feel empowered. That's because losing weight is nothing to be ashamed of, it should be admired.

That's why I strongly suggest that the minute that you embark on the last leg of this book, you get the help of a friend or other loved one to keep you on track. If athletes have coaches to push them to do their best, why shouldn't you have the same thing in your life?

"Coaching" could prove to be invaluable. A friend/coach could be that phone call that keeps your cravings in check and your weight loss on track. Best of all, if you are both in this together, you can be the same for them if you both give it a chance. Every little bit helps.

As you embark on this journey, don't feel afraid to tell anyone that you are eating healthier. I do. They will realize it when they see your significant weight loss. They will notice your new wardrobe or that you are finally wearing clothes that you haven't worn in years. But, even then, remember that this weight loss is for you.

But, just don't use the word "diet." The word "diet" has such a bad reputation and some people will be tempted to help you break it or cheat on it. Instead, watch the look on a person's face the next time that they suggest you have a piece of cheesecake for dessert and you reveal that you are trying to eat healthier. Nine times out of ten, they will ask for your secret, and then, to join you.

By telling your co-workers, family and friends, you will also increase your accountability, especially if you have children. By making the decision to eat healthier, you are setting the tone for your entire family to follow.

If you are a parent or plan to become one, it is your responsibility to provide the right food for your family, planning your meals and eliminating distractions at the dinner table. The biggest problem is that your children's eating habits can be one of the biggest barriers your losing weight. The worst part is that you already know it.

Right now, you are probably wondering how? You should know that the only responsibility of a child is to eat or not to eat. But, in most families, the child is often the one who decides what to eat. Sure your child may love macaroni and cheese with no vegetables, or even, often hot dogs. What happens when you find yourself eating it too? Where is the nutrition in that?

As a child, you may have often had to probably eat what was served, or wait until the next meal. Now, as an adult, you feel like you wouldn't ever do this to yourself or your child. You won't force anyone to eat what they don't want, or when they don't want to. Would you?

When you force anyone to eat, you are robbing them, especially children, of developing a natural ability to determine if they are still hungry or naturally full. This is intuitive eating. Yet, the irony of it all is that you will do this to yourself most days. You will still eat what, when and how it is expected of you, which leads to poor eating habits and poor weight management

Why? As children, we weren't always taught that we needed to eat healthier. As teens, because of this we just ate what we wanted when we wanted. Now as we set out to be a good example or role model in our eating for others, especially our children, we have to fortify our own resolve to eat healthier first.

Teach your children, friends and family now that fad dieting doesn't maintain your weight, healthy eating does. With healthy eating, you aren't just losing weight, you are adding years to your life. Years that you could spend enjoying your life, your hobbies and your family.

You should know that there is always going to be someone who will tell you that you shouldn't have to diet. When they say this, thank them, or say "how sweet," and then, move on. This weight loss again is about you. You shouldn't have to justify why you are trying to eat healthier. You want to look better. You want to eat better. You want to feel better. You want to have more energy. You want to lose weight.

The key is to maintain this motivation, even if it means choosing a picture of you when you were at your heaviest and put it up where you can see it every day with a note with your goal written where you can see that too. If your goal is to lose 20 pounds, post the picture and write right next to it, "I will lose 20 pounds and end up weighing 135." But, how?

You can do this, and right now, there is only one thing left to do. Let's start eating healthier. I'm not going to not only show you how to do it, I am going to show you how much and why you should be doing it...

What Your Day Should Look Like...

So now that we know what good calories look like, how to get the good fat and cholesterol that we need and the right amount of servings to eat. Let's talk about what your day should look like...

The key to losing weight for you right now is making sure that you have the right balance of carbs in your diet. To do this, just like water, we need to know how much we need to survive each day.

Despite what other diet plans will tell you, your goal right now is to get your weight back to your ideal weight, which is the amount of weight that you were born to have, regardless if it is a size six or a size twelve. Why even try to fool with Mother Nature?

With a little math using the Harris-Benedict principle to calculate your Basal Metabolic Rate, or BMR, we can determine the right amount of calories that you will need to live and to perform basic functions, such as breathing.

Using this simple formula, which you can do on a calculator, or even on the calculator that you have on your phone, you can then determine the amount of calories that you need to maintain your ideal weight.

By consuming the right amount of carbs, you will begin to see a significant weight loss. This is also the secret to keeping that weight off for good. So, let's begin...step one, ladies, is to calculate your BMR, with the following formula. Please note that this formula is for and should only be used by adults.

If you are using your phone calculator and it doesn't have all the bells and whistles of a regular calculator, don't worry. I will now go a little slower. Let's start...Multiply your ideal weight; the weight that we determined on page 45, which you should know by heart, by 4.3 to find your weight score. Write that number down.

Ideal Weight   Times Factor   Equals   Weight Score

_____   X   4.35   =   _____

Then, I need you to multiply your height in inches, by 4.7 to find your height score. One foot equals 12 inches. If you are, let's say, 5' 2", or five feet two inches, 12 times 5 equals 60. Then, plus the 2 is 62. It sounds simple, but we all have been out of school for some time. You should multiply your height times 4.7, and then, write that number down.

Height   Times Factor Equals   Height Score

_____   X   4.7   =   _____

Next, take your age and multiple that by 4.7 to find your age score. Write that number down.

Age   Times   Factor   Equals   Age Score

_____   X   4.3   =   _____

Now, add 655 plus your weight score. Next, add your height score to that. Then, subtract your age score. You now have your BMR.

Starting Point (the 655 number) + Weight Score + Height Score – Age Score = Basal Metabolic Rate

Your BMR number is _____.

Stay with me! This just the first step, but it is very important. Now, we need to get really honest. In order to know how many calories that you will be able to eat every day. So let's begin, ask yourself, this…how active are you in your daily life? Please be honest.

Are you sedentary? Do you have a job or a lifestyle that requires you to sit down a lot or do you have limited movement? Then, multiple your BMR number by 1.2 percent. This number is the number of calories you should consume every day and that number is _____.

Are you lightly active? Do you have a job or a lifestyle that allows you the opportunity to exercise 1 to 3 days a week? Then, multiple your BMR number by 1.375. This number is the number of calories you should consume every day and that number is _____.

Are you moderately active? Do you have a job or a lifestyle that allows you the opportunity to move around a lot or you exercise 3 to 5 days per week? Then, multiple your BMR number by 1.4. This number is the number of calories you should consume every day and that number is _____.

Are you very active? Do you have a job or a lifestyle that allows you to exercise for longer periods or 6 to 7 days per week? Then, multiple your BMR number by 1.75. This number is the number of calories you should consume every day and that number is _____.

Now, let's put it all together. In order to reach your ideal weight. You now have your ideal weight, your water intake amount, and lastly, your suggested caloric intake level, courtesy of your Basal Metabolic Rate, or BMR.

So let's say that you are five feet four inches tall and you are 30 years old. You currently weigh 155 pounds and using the ideal weight chart, you figured out that your body is really a medium frame and that your ideal weight is between 124 and 138 pounds.

That means your goal should be to lose about 20 pounds. You should then set a goal to attempt to lose up to two pounds a week. This should take you about 12 weeks or three months, barring any issues.

You have had a physical and you don't have any issues barring you from increasing your water intake every day. So now, you divided your weight by two and determined that you need to be drinking about 75 ounces of water every day. That's about 10 cups. That's it. That's all.

But, wait, it's not enough to just eat the right amount of calories. You need to know how many calories are also in certain foods. Let's take some of the guess work out of figuring out how many calories are in your favorite foods. Don't be afraid to use this book as a cheat sheet until you know how to take an educated guess...

Your One Stop Guide To Calories

It's good to know how many calories that you are consuming whether you are on a diet or just making sure that you are eating enough to stay healthy.

That's why I have put together a list of several common foods and how many calories that you can expect to find in each serving or portion. This way you can keep track of your caloric intake every day.

A calorie is something that you need to be aware of as you lose weight. The slimmer your body, the fewer calories that you will eventually need to maintain that weight. Also, you should also never feel hungry again.

Also, if you decide to have a beer (144 calories) with your co-workers or friends after work, you won't berate yourself up for it. It simply means that you will have to be inspired to work it off some other way. Go do the dishes or some laundry, which actually helps to burn off calories! Yes, doing dishes and laundry helps.

Also remember that there are a lot of great low calorie substitutes for high calorie foods, such as a chicken burger (130 calories) versus a hamburger (250 calories). You just have to look!

The goal right now is to end this love-hate relationship that most people have with counting calories in order to lose weight. You should also know that I am not going to make you even try to count every last calorie. The key is awareness about how many calories certain foods have in them. Aware is key and awareness brings about change in how and what you eat.

For example, if you know that you should only consume 2,000 calories day, then, an eight ounce steak alone will account for about 700 calories. Bake two lamb chops (256 calories) and have a cup of broccoli (24) with an ounce of cheddar cheese (114), pasta (100) and a cup of tea with honey (110). That's only 606 calories.

Those 606 calories sounds a lot better than one 700 calorie steak that you haven't even added a side to or a vegetable. Then, don't forget the steak sauce or your gravy. That's a lot of calories. That's calories and more calories that your body really doesn't need.

You should also know that these caloric suggestions aren't written in stone, it is okay to go slightly over your limit of a 600 calorie dinner, but, not too far though. When in doubt, don't eat it. If it is not good for you, you are not being good to you.

Remember that a healthy meal will keep you within your limit and on track to your ideal weight and a healthier you. At this point, with all calories, awareness is key. Again, awareness brings about change...

Meats	Portion	Calories
Raw Beef	1 ounce	88
Raw Lean Beef	1 ounce	75
Grilled/Broiled Beef	1 ounce	107
Lamb	1 ounce	80
Lamb Chop	1 chop	128

Deer	1 ounce	42
Pepperoni	1 ounce	148
Grilled/Broiled Steak	1 ounce	51
Raw Bacon	1 ounce	150
Cooked Bacon	1 ounce	135
Ham	1 ounce	45
Pork	1 ounce	76
Pork Chop	1 ounce	75
Pork Sausage	1 patty	92
Pork Roast	1 ounce	55
Chicken Roasted	1 cup	240
Chicken Hot dog	1 full	116
Turkey	1 ounce	45
Turkey Dogtrot	1 full	102
Caviar	1 ounce	72
Raw Clams	1 medium	11
Canned Clams	1 cup	237
Cod	1 ounce	25
Crab	1 ounce	30
Lobster	1 ounce	33
Raw Oyster	1 medium	8
Salmon	1 ounce	50
Canned Salmon	1 ounce	40

Raw Scallops	1 ounce	25
Shrimp	1 ounce	30
Prawns	1 ounce	30
Tuna	1 ounce	50
Canned Tuna	1 ounce	35

Vegetables	Serving	Calories
Red Pepper	1 medium	39
Green Pepper	1 medium	17
Small Potato	1 medium	88
Baked Potato	1 medium	161
Baked Sweet Potato	1 medium	136
Boiled Potato	1 medium	861
Fresh Potato	1 medium	80
Cucumber	1 medium	19
Raw Asparagus	1 ounce	8
Fresh Green Beans	1 cup	44
Canned Green Beans	1 cup	46
Beetroot	1 cup	60
Broccoli	1 cup	24
Brussels Sprouts	1 ounce	12
Raw Cabbage	1 cup	56

Corn	1 cup	132
Raw Eggplant	1 medium	27
Garlic	1 clove	4
Ginger	1 ounce	20
Saffron	1 teaspoon	2
Salt	1 teaspoon	0
Lettuce	1 head	21
Mushrooms	1 cup	20
White Onion	1 medium	40
Green Onions	1 cup	32
Canned Pumpkin	1 cup	80
Radish	1 cup	18
Raw Spinach	1 leaf	2
Tomato	1 medium	26
Fresh Green Beans	1 cup	44
Green Peas	1 cup	96
Shallots	1 tablespoon	8
Tomatillo	1 medium	11

Fruits	Portion	Calories
Apple	1 medium	80
Apricot	1 medium	17
Avocado	1 ounce	50

Banana	1 medium	105
Blackberries	1 cup	74
Blueberries	1 cup	82
Boysenberries	1 cup	82
Fresh Cherries	1 cup	100
Dried Cherries	1 cup	560
Cantaloupe	1 medium	188
Cranberries	1 cup	46
Dates	1 cup	502
Fig	1 medium	37
Dried Figs	5 figs	240
Grapes	1 cup	62
Grapefruit	1 medium	120
Kiwifruit	1 medium	46
Lemon	1 medium	17
Lime	1 medium	20
Mango	1 medium	135
Nectarine	1 medium	67
Orange	1 medium	62
Papaya	1 medium	117
Peach	1 medium	37
Pear	1 medium	100

Canned Pear	1 ounce	75
Pineapple	1 cup	78
Plum	1 ounce	16
Pomegranate	1 ounce	19
Raisins	1 cup	438
Strawberries	1 cup	46
Tangerine	1 medium	37
Watermelon	1 cup	50

Other Foods	Portion	Calories
Bread	1 slice	70
Cornflakes	1 cup	100
Cheddar Cheese	1 ounce	114
Cottage Cheese	1 cup	234
Tofu	1 ounce	22
Chocolate	1 ounce	140
White Chocolate	1 ounce	162
Dark Chocolate	1 ounce	180
Cocoa	1 cup	200
Cornstarch	1 tablespoon	30
Ketchup	1 tablespoon	15
Mayonnaise	1 tablespoon	100

Mustard	1 tablespoon	10
Olive	1 full	12
Oatmeal	1 cup	145
Chocolate Syrup	1 tablespoon	25
Yeast	1 ounce	80
Soy Sauce	1 tablespoon	11
Buttermilk	1 cup	100
Soy Milk	1 cup	80
Greek Yogurt	1 cup	140
Egg	1 full	75
Butter	1 tablespoon	100
Peanut Butter	1 tablespoon	95
Almonds	1 ounce	160
Cashews	1 ounce	160
Peanuts	1 ounce	160
Walnuts	1 ounce	140
Pistachios	1 ounce	165
Barley	1 cup	650
Noodles	1 cup	190
Cream of Tartar	1 teaspoon	2
Popcorn	1 ounce	110
Salsa	1 tablespoon	3
Pasta	1 ounce	100

Rice	1 cup	240
Brown Rice	1 cup	210
Honey	1 tablespoon	60
Maple Syrup	1 tablespoon	50

Beverage	Serving Size	Calories
Milk	1 cup	157
Beer	1 bottle	144
Gin	1 ounce	65
Rum	1 ounce	65
Vodka	1 ounce	65
Whiskey	1 ounce	65
Red Wine	1 ounce	23
White Wine	1 ounce	22
Coffee	1 cup	40
Tea	1 cup	50

In addition to being aware of the calories, we have to make these words a part of your everyday vocabulary: baked, boiled, broiled, dry broiled (in lemon juice or wine,) garden fresh, grilled, high fiber, in its own juice, poached, red sauce, roasted, steamed and whole grain. These words will make every one of your meals better. Speaking of meals, let's talk about a new meal plan...

Finally, A Meal Plan That You Can Live With...

Now that we know about calories, if you really want to keep it simple, now that you know your BMR, or the amount of calories that you need to reach your ideal or goal weight, take that number and divide it by five. That's the number of small meals that you could eat, instead of three meals and two snacks.

For instance, let's say that you need 2000 calories, divided by those 2000 calories into five. You can then eat five meals of about 400 calories. (2500 then that's 500 calories that you can have per meal.) I would never recommend anyone going below 2000 calories per day. It is just not healthy or safe.

If 2000 calories is all that you need, you can simply use the United Stated Department of Health And Human Services and the United States Department Of Agriculture's guideline for a 2000 calorie day:

- ✓ 300-500 calorie breakfast
- ✓ 150 calorie snack
- ✓ 400-600 calorie lunch
- ✓ 150 calorie snack
- ✓ 400-600 calorie dinner

Knowing this will also help you order at many restaurants that are required to, or voluntarily, list their calories on the menu, like Subway. Also, if you know that what you are eating is over the required calories, then, eat it while drinking a glass of water. Water doesn't have any calories to add to your caloric intake.

So here is a week of the Department of Agriculture recommended menu for a 2000 calorie diet. Feel free to remove the things that you don't like and add the things that you do. This is just a suggestion...

DAY ONE:

BREAKFAST:
Breakfast burrito
- Take 1 flour tortilla (7" diameter)
- Scramble 1 organic egg (in macadamia nut oil)
- Add 1/3 cup of cooked black beans
- Add 2 tablespoons of salsa
1 cup orange juice
1 cup fat-free milk

LUNCH:

Roast beef sandwich
- Split 1 whole grain sandwich bun
- Add 3 ounces of lean roast beef
- Add 2 slices of tomato
- Add 1/4 cup shredded romaine lettuce
- Add 1/8 cup of mushrooms (sautéed in 1 teaspoons of toasted sesame oil)
- Add 1 1/2 ounce part-skim mozzarella cheese
- Add 1 teaspoon yellow mustard
On the side 3/4 cup of baked potato chips
1 unsweetened beverage

DINNER

Stuffed broiled salmon
- Using 2 teaspoons of canola oil, rub salmon with oil and use the rest to oil your broiler

- Prepare 1/2 cup saffron or jasmine rice
- Steam 1/2 cup of broccoli, season with a seasoning
  like Mrs. Dash to your taste
- Add up to one teaspoon of olive oil spread
1 teaspoons of olive oil spread
1 cup fat-free milk

SNACK IDEAS:

1 cup of cantaloupe or honey dew

Day Two:

BREAKFAST:

Hot cereal (oatmeal, cream of wheat)
- Prepare 1/2 cup of oatmeal
- Add 2 tablespoons raisins
- Season with raw sugar to your taste level
1/2 cup of fat-free milk
1 cup of orange juice

LUNCH:

Taco salad
- Add 2 ounces of tortilla chips
- Add 2 ounces of sautéed ground turkey,
- Add 1/2 cup of black beans, canned but drained to
  remove excess salt, is okay
- Add 1/2 cup of iceberg lettuce
- Add 2 slices of tomato
- Add 1 ounce of low-fat cheddar cheese
- Add 2 tablespoons of salsa

- Add 1/2 cup of avocado
- Add 1 teaspoon of lime juice and mix ingredients
1 unsweetened beverage, like water

DINNER

Spinach lasagna,
- Boil 1 cup of lasagna noodles
- Assembled in layers with the following
- 2/3 cup of cooked spinach
- 1/2 cup of ricotta cheese
- 1/2 cup of tomato sauce tomato bits
- 1 ounce of part-skim mozzarella cheese
- Bake for 30 minutes until cheese has melted
1 whole wheat dinner roll
1 cup of fat-free milk

SNACK IDEAS:

1/2 ounce of dry-roasted almonds
1/4 cup of pineapple
2 tablespoons of raisins

Day Three:

BREAKFAST:

Cold cereal
- 1 cup of Honey Nut (or other flavors) Cheerios
- 1 cup of fat-free milk
- 1 small banana
1 slice of whole wheat toast
- 1 teaspoon of olive oil spread

1 cup of prune juice (it is good for you)

LUNCH:

Tuna fish sandwich
- Using 2 slices of honey wheat bread
- Mix 3 ounces of tuna (packed in water and drained)
- Add 2 teaspoons of mayonnaise
- Add 1 tablespoon of diced celery and mix
- Spread mixture on bread
- Add 1/4 cup of shredded romaine lettuce
- Add 2 slices of tomato
1 medium pear
1 cup of fat-free milk

DINNER

Roasted chicken breast
- Seasoned and broiled 3 ounces of boneless skinless chicken breast with Mrs. Dash for 1 hour at 350 degree
- Bake 1 large sweet potato with your chicken and serve with pepper and olive oil spread
- On the stove, prepare 1/2 cup peas and diced onions
- Add 1 teaspoon of olive oil spread
1 whole wheat dinner roll
Prepare 1 cup of leafy greens salad
- Add lite salad dressing of your choice

SNACK IDEAS:

1/4 cup of dried apricots or peaches
1 cup of low-fat fruited yogurt

Day Four:

BREAKFAST:

1 whole wheat English muffin
- 2 teaspoons of olive oil spread
- 1 tablespoon of jam or preserves
1 medium grapefruit
1 hard-boiled egg
1 unsweetened beverage

LUNCH:

White bean-vegetable soup
- 1 1/4 cup of chunky vegetable soup
- 1/2 cup of cooked white beans
2 ounces bread stick
8 baby carrots
1 cup of fat-free milk

DINNER

Rigatoni with meat sauce
- Boil 1 cup of rigatoni pasta and drain
 - Add 1/2 cup of chunky spaghetti sauce
 - Add 2 ounces extra lean cooked ground beef (sautéed in 2 teaspoons vegetable oil)
 - Season to your taste with sugar (yes, sugar)
 - Serve with grated Parmesan cheese
Tossed spinach salad with:
- 1 cup of baby spinach leaves
- 1/2 cup of tangerine slices
- 1/2 ounce of chopped walnuts
- 3 teaspoons of sunflower oil and vinegar dressing
1 cup of fat-free milk

SNACK IDEAS:

1 cup of low-fat fruited yogurt

Day FIVE:

BREAKFAST:

Cold cereal
- 1 cup of flavored multi-grain cereal
- 1 tablespoon of raisins
- 1 cup of fat-free milk
- 1 small banana
1 slice of whole wheat toast
- 1 teaspoon of olive oil spread
- 1 teaspoon of jelly

LUNCH:

Smoked turkey sandwich
- Using 2 ounces of whole wheat pita bread
- Add 1/4 cup of romaine lettuce
- Add 2 slices of tomato
- Add 3 ounces of sliced smoked turkey breast
- Add 1 tablespoon of mayo-type salad dressing
- Add 1 teaspoon of yellow mustard
1/2 cup of apple slices
1 cup of tomato juice or V8 fruit juice

DINNER

Grilled top loin steak

- Using toasted sesame seed oil, brown a 5 ounces top loin steak that has been marinated, and then, cook at low temperature until tender, seasoned to your taste
Prepare 3/4 cups of mashed potatoes
- Add 2 teaspoons of olive oil spread and pepper
Steam 1/2 cup of carrots
- Add 1 tablespoon of honey
2 ounces whole wheat dinner roll
- Add 1 teaspoon of olive oil spread
1 cup of fat-free milk

SNACK IDEAS:

1 cup of low-fat fruited yogurt

DAY SIX:

BREAKFAST:

French toast
- Using 2 slices of whole wheat bread
- Mix three organic eggs, a quarter cup of fat free milk and cinnamon.
- Coat bread with mixture
- Using 2 teaspoons of macadamia nut oil, brown both slices of each piece of bread
- Serve with 2 tablespoons of maple syrup
1/2 medium grapefruit
1 cup of fat-free milk

LUNCH:

Vegetarian chili on baked potato

- Bake on large potato
- Split potato and add vegetarian chili onto potato
- Add 1 ounce of low fat cheddar cheese and serve
1/2 cup of cantaloupe
3/4 cup of lemonade

DINNER

Hawaiian pizza
- Using 2 slices of cheese pizza
- Top with 1 ounce of cooked Canadian bacon
- Add 1/4 cup of pineapple
- Add 2 tablespoons of mushrooms
- Add 2 tablespoons of chopped onions
- Prepare according to pizza directions and serve
Green salad
- Add 1 cup of leafy greens, like spinach
- Add 3 teaspoons of balsamic vinaigrette
1 cup fat-free milk

SNACK IDEAS:

5 whole wheat crackers
1/8 cup of hummus
1/2 cup of fruit cocktail (in water or juice)

DAY SEVEN:

BREAKFAST:

Pancakes
- Prepare 3 buttermilk pancakes using macadamia nut
  oil to grease your pan as directed

- Serve with maple syrup
1/2 cup of strawberries
3/4 cup of honeydew melon
1/2 cup of fat-free milk

LUNCH:

Manhattan clam chowder
10 whole wheat crackers
1 medium orange
1 cup of fat-free milk

DINNER

Eat what you choose
1 cup of lemon-flavored iced tea

SNACK IDEAS:

1 ounce of sunflower seeds
1 large banana
1 cup of low-fat fruited yogurt

Again, feel free to change whatever you don't like. Just use the calorie guide to make better choices. Food doesn't have to be bland, it should be proportionally correct though. After you eat, answer this question for me, how do you feel? Full? Bloated? There is only one answer...

How Should You Feel After You Eat?

After you eat, you should always feel better. You should never feel stuffed, bloated, or even, tired. Remember, your stomach is the size of a fist; you only need a hand full of something to fill it comfortably.

When it comes to snacks, be choosy about what you eat. The other rule is to not eat anything after dinner. The next meal that you should have is breakfast, the next day. Again, children are smart, at night many of them ask for a glass of water and this helps curb their hunger, use it to your advantage to control your hunger.

A good teacher will lead you to what they want you to see, but they won't tell you what to look at. So choose you meals carefully, be mindful of the salt. Be mindful also of the fat and the calories. Every meal should include something from the four major food groups whenever possible: dairy, meat, grains and fruits and vegetables. Your snacks should contain at least two.

So let's say that you are planning dinner, because that's what we do now. You might have salmon, which is a meat and it is filled with good protein, brown rice which serves as a grain, with a side of baby carrots, which is your veggie and a glass of milk, which is your dairy.

For lunch, let's say you had a slice of pizza. This works when it is a slice of pizza with let's say ground beef. The crust is the grain. The cheese is the dairy. The beef is the protein, which is another example of something that you don't have to have a lot of meat to enjoy it and benefit from it. The sauce is the fruit and if you added let's say peppers and onions, you have it all.

In order to avoid relying on fast food, try to also to learn to cook for the week or the night before put something in the oven that you can heat and eat later. Whenever possible, make sure it is fresh. The last thing you want to feel is that nasty rebound hunger.

You should know that this rebound hunger stems from eating out of can. Yes, the same canned goods that you depend on because they are quick and easy to prepare can leave you feeling hungry. Yes, that same quick canned pasta or soup. Forget about the salt intake for a minute. Ask yourself, when was the last time that you ate out of a can? There is something there that you should be concerned about.

It is the chemical bisphenol A, or BPA. BPA is the same chemical, which they removed from all baby bottles because of the health risk when they are heated. This is the same chemical is in most canned goods. BPA is in the lining that seals the cans of most foods.

For most foods, it's safe, but what about highly acidic foods, like tomato paste? There is a concern that this chemical can leak into your food. Why should you be concerned? BPA has been linked to some problems in babies and children, and prostate problems in men.

According to the Federal Food and Drug Administration or the FDA, this same chemical, BPA, that manufacturers use to preserve a food's shelf life, also raises the leptin levels in your body, making you think that you are still hungry.

Leptin is an influential hormone, or protein, in the body that is produced by human fat cells. What Leptin does in the body is to tell the brain how much fat is stored in the body. It controls your appetite, energy levels, hormone balance and your metabolism. Leptin is essential for survival; it guides your body's proper response to hunger. Essentially, Leptin helps control your weight.

When you are lean and have very little fat stored, leptin helps to regulate your weight by controlling appetite and the use of stored energy. However, if you are overweight and there is a problem with the leptin levels, then, trouble occurs.

This could be the primary reason for food cravings, overeating, an obsession with food, and a slow metabolism. Overweight individuals appear to be resistant to leptin, similar to diabetic people being resistant to insulin. That's why you should always check with your doctor before starting any diet and always have a complete physical, like I suggested.

The problem for most people is that BPA is always giving them a false message of hunger, or rebound hunger, and their metabolism reacts to this, even when food and body fat is already abundant. So, eat fresh whenever possible, to avoid BPA, especially with tomato based foods, likes sauces or canned pasta. It is better for you.

As you are reading this book now, what are you doing? Hopefully, you are not eating or snacking. In order to learn how to eat healthier, we also need to fight our cravings for what we used to think of as comfort food...

If Those Chips Or Cookies Aren't Your Husband, Then, They Shouldn't Be In Your Bedroom...

I love Snickers candy bars. What is even worse than that is that I love snicker doodle cookies. I love them. But, by ending my destructive relationship with food, I loved them enough to let them go. That's what you do with any bad relationship, you two break up. The question is "Can you still be friends?" The answer is yes!

Remember that dieting doesn't mean deprivation. You shouldn't have to give up everything that you love. You just can't always have them every time that you want or as much as you want. You have to learn to fight your cravings with everything that you have. A nap. A glass of water. A long walk. A phone call. Sugar free gum.

If you feel like you are going to cheat, be prepared to deal with it with something other than anger, resentment or guilt. Accept that it happened, forgive yourself and keep going. Sure, you might have eaten a whole candy bar, but it is not the end of the world.

Remember that when you can't fight your cravings, use moderation. Practice the rule of one. You can have one cookie and a large glass of water, but you can't have the cookie unless you finish the water, which will curb your cravings for more cookies. You might not even want the cookie then. This is a good thing.

Remember that certain foods will always be tempting, like Grandmother's cake that you ate growing up. For some things, they have become more habit than what is truly good for you. You have to minimalize their hold on you. I have been in the supermarket and had the Red

Velvet Cake call my name. Like a bill collector or your annoying cousin, you don't have to answer their call.

Also, avoid habits that produce cravings like excessive TV commercials and cooking shows. We love them, but usually the person cooking, like Rachel Ray, is cute and thin. I stopped watching her. She left me feeling hungry. The only person that I watch cook now is me.

At certain times, the kitchen should be off limit. Put a sign up that at 8 o'clock the kitchen is closed. It is. How many times have you wandered in there only to end up eating something that you don't need or you really didn't want? After 8 is too late. Remember that!

You will only end up with an arm full of goodies going back to the couch or your bedroom. You might end up feeling too lazy to put back the rest, so you eat all of it. For those moments, I stock up on impulse meals like fruit and I keep it readily available. Or find the fat-free equivalent, like popcorn or baked potato chips.

If I leave a bowl of fruit on the table in the dining room, like oranges, then I stop myself from going into the kitchen to eat something that is not good for me. No dining room? Leave a bowl of sugar free candy in the living room on the table. It works for your grandmother.

Often, if I want something, I will tell myself that I can have it on Friday. This gives me something to look forward to during a long week. When Friday comes, nine times out of ten, I have forgotten all about it. Speaking of forgetting, there is one thing you should never forget. Curious? Good. It's called exercise...

Now, Lift Those Legs And One, Two...What?

To me, exercising is like fighting a bear. It is not something that I ever thought that I could win. But, who says that bear has to be a grizzly bear. What if that "bear" turned out to a koala bear? That's why when it comes to exercise you have to figure out what works for you, and then, make it work for you. It doesn't matter if you walk, jog or run. You have to get moving.

Add some kind of exercise to your daily life. The key is to not overdo it. You will only find yourself saying "I am tired. I don't feel like working out today because I exercised a lot yesterday." With proper exercise, you won't actually feel so tired. Exercise actually improves your sleep habits. It helps fight fatigue. It will also help you to manage your stress.

The one thing that a specific exercise can't do is to tone a specific part of the body. Exercise peels back the layers of your whole body like an onion. If you want a flatter belly, or to lose the flab on your arms, you have to move your whole body, not just do sit ups.

The first step is to know that it doesn't have to be something extravagant, it just has to be doable. Don't over think it. If you over think it, you will give yourself so many reasons why you can't do it. Get moving. Again, you can walk, jog or run. Just do it.

To get yourself going, again, doesn't have to be hard. It can be as simple as taking your children, or a niece or a nephew, to the playground and not just sitting down and watching them, go play with them. Who says that you can't? Get out there and show them.

You should also know that I get so tired of hearing people say that they don't have 30 minutes to fit into their busy schedule to work out. Yet, every night, you spend at least two hours in front of the television set wondering why you can't lose weight. If you take care of your body, it will take care of you.

Also, the craziest thing that I have ever heard is that you can't exercise until you lose weight. What? Who told you that? You can exercise at any weight. It is the key to maintaining your weight loss after you have lost the weight, but, you also can't lose any weight without it.

Most people when they find something that they like, they stick to it. But, the truth is you have to change it up to see real results. Yes, you like to walk, but how about going out for a night of dancing? How about taking an aerobics class or buying an aerobics DVD to work out to? Get moving. It doesn't matter how you do it. Just do it.

Also, you can never just exercise. Eating anything that you want, and then, trying to run it off afterwards will not work. Dieting and exercise comes in pairs. You have to work at both to see the results that you want.

When you do get active, stay active. Remember when I talked about the people who never seem to gain a pound, they are still childlike in their approach. They keep moving. For everything that they think that they shouldn't have eaten, like that piece of cake, they find a way to work it off. It may be subconscious, but they do it.

Believe it or not, spontaneous physical activity, like doing laundry, or even the dishes, can burn up to 350 calories a day. That's why I hinted at it before. It is what my brother does. He is a teacher and he drinks a 20 ounce Mountain Dew soda every single day. Sure, it is loaded with empty calories and added sugar, but during his day he often walks up and down three flights of stairs, at least 12 times a day. He has never liked bread, doesn't drink whole milk and he maintains his weight.

The key to any exercise is to find a way to fit it into your life, and then, find the motivation to get it done. Don't be afraid to mix it up. Do one thing, one day and something else on the others. Here is a list of just some of the things that you can do:

✓ Walking	✓ Jumping rope
✓ Running	✓ Roller skating
✓ Dancing	✓ Bike riding
✓ Doing Aerobics	✓ Playing Tennis
✓ Water aerobics	✓ Basketball
✓ Swimming	✓ Bowling

Most days, even I don't feel like working out. If the problem is that you don't have the time. You can make time for everyone else, why not you? Eating healthier plus exercise will give you the edge.

The key is finding a work out partner. Remember, I said to get help, I meant it. You will need it. You will then work harder and this coaching will push you farther. Time goes by faster when you have somebody with you. If you can't find a partner, but you have children, take your children with you. They can use the exercise too.

Your children, or niece or nephew, can ride a bike or their skates as you walk along. If you love to ride a bike or skates, do it. Nobody ever said that you have to turn into a fitness instructor to lose weight.

If you don't have children, or a workout partner, make a play list of your favorite music to match your activity. Play the music at a comfortable level, so that you can hear the traffic or sense danger and always walk in a well-lit and well-populated area only. Always place your safety over your fitness plans.

Ten songs could give you a good thirty minute workout. The faster the beat, the more motivated you will be. You can even do this when cleaning the house. It works. Also, don't be afraid to tell the world about it. Post your successes and not your failures on Facebook: "Hey, just walked five miles and I feel great." Watch the accolades roll in. Someone may want to join you the next time.

Remember that picture of the old you with the note that reminds you of your goal, use it as your motivation. Remember can't means won't! You will only then begin to believe what you tell yourself if you say that you can't do it. If you say that you can't lose weight, you won't. Remember that your goal is to look better, feel better, eat better and have more energy too.

The goal is to get your heart rate going. You want to increase your heart rate. You want to increase your breathing through a cardio workout, like walking, jogging, running, or even, swimming. This is what a cardiovascular workout is all about. Don't be afraid to work up a sweat. That is just your fat crying tears!

Cardio means "heart" and vascular is about the blood vessels that carry blood to and from the heart. When you increase your breathing, you increase the amount of oxygen that your body takes in, which also helps to strengthen your cardiovascular system. Did you know that by getting your cardiovascular system going, you are also boosting your mood? Chances are you will feel much better after a workout.

The one thing that you don't want to do is to overdo it. This might actually backfire on you. When you overdo it, your body will work harder to stay in balance. Your body may respond by cuing your body to eat more. When you eat more, you are sabotaging your weight loss efforts.

Surprise your body with intervals of high intensity activity. This could be as simple as getting off the train, maybe the stop before your job, and if it is safe and you have the time, try walking the rest of the way to work.

Or if you drive, park away from the entrance at the far end of the parking lot and you, then, walk the rest of the way. Once there, you can walk the last five flights up to your office, rather than taking the elevator. Whatever you do, get moving and keep moving.

Look at your daily schedule and figure out the best time that you can do this. It should always be with few distractions. Also, monitor your sleep activities afterward. If you know you will be wide awake, don't exercise before bed time. If you know you will feel tired afterwards, then right before bedtime might be the best time to exercise. Proper sleep is very important.

With any exercise, just do it, and then, stick to it. Even if you miss a day, keep going. What you will learn is that this exercise coupled with better food choices will help you lose all of the weight that you need to lose, and then, permanently keep it off. Remember your exercise routine doesn't have to come with an expensive gym membership. You can burn up to 100 calories or more simply by doing more of what you do every day. Including...

- ✓ A brisk walk is the easiest way to burn calories. If you notice cities, like New York, where people walk more, they tend to be thinner.
- ✓ Dancing. Just 20 minutes of those dance video games or a night out dancing at your local club will help burn off the calories too.
- ✓ Can't go out running, remember in gym class, when the teachers made you jog in place, try it now. Give it your best for 10 minutes.
- ✓ Vacuuming and cleaning your floors for just a half an hour will burn calories.
- ✓ Housework, like ironing clothes will burn the calories off. You have to do it any way, why not lose weight while you do it.
- ✓ Remember when I said about taking the stairs at work. You don't have to walk up twenty flights, but you can do five, or even, ten flights. Try it on your way home. Walk down the stairs.
- ✓ New Moms? Take a walk with your new baby. Your child will love it and your body will too. Your baby will also sleep so much better.

Again, the bottom line is even if you can't "exercise," get moving. You can do it. If it is important to you, you will find a way. If not, you will find an excuse, stop making excuses and just do it, and then, stay motivated to keep doing it, even when you don't feel like it...

Weighing In And Staying Motivated!

Should you or should you not keep track of your weight? How else will you know if you don't weigh in? Always, do it without clothing and in the morning. If you did it at night, you might not always like what you see, which can destroy your motivation to lose weight.

By staying motivated, even during your weigh in, you will definitely see the results. But, you must set your goal and stick to it. Make your weigh in a part of your daily goals and stay motivated to do it, just like you check your email or Facebook page.

You ideal or goal weight is where you want to be in your weight loss efforts. Every day, take the time to say this aloud to yourself.

I want to look better.

I want to eat better.

I want to feel better.

I want to have more energy.

I am losing the weight!

I can do this.

Write this down, type it up, and then, print it out. Sign your name and post it up wherever you need to, so that you can see it. Put the proverbial carrot in front of the horse and wagon and get moving on where you want to be. This is not for me. It is for you.

You are your biggest cheerleader. Sometimes, it helps to hear something good from somebody who knows you best. Who knows you better than you? It also will help replace a lot of your negative thoughts about yourself and fight those fears of what you can't do when it comes to reaching your ideal weight. You can do this!

If a pair of your favorite jeans don't fit, don't buy a new pair of jeans, do what you need to do to get back into your old pairs. Hang those jeans where you can see it and say to yourself, I will fit those jeans again. Let that be your motivation. Your body will follow your lead.

When you do lose that first ten pounds, make sure that you reward yourself, but not with food. Let wearing those jeans again be your reward.

Or how about this, for every pound that you lose, put a dollar, or even five dollars, in a jar? When you have reached your goal, buy yourself something new to wear to go along with those jeans to celebrate. You have earned this reward.

Now, my friend, here comes the not so easy part of all of this, let's learn to keep track of your progress, both the highs and the lows. The highs, or successes, will tell you what works and the lows, or the failures, will show you what does not work for you.

No weight loss system should ever be without this step. How else will you know what you are capable of? You have to track your success. Let me show you how…

Here Comes The Not So Hard Part...
Keeping Track Of Your Results

On the following pages, I have provided several pages to allow you to keep track of the foods that you eat and how you will eat for the next week. You might not want to tote this book around, so simply writing it down, and then, adding it to the book later is fine.

Lately, I have been making it easier than even that, I simply texted myself a message. It only takes a minute. With this tracking system, I want you to keep track of how much you weigh every day. Yes, every day. You can do it. You will need to see the results.

Also, never get discouraged by what you find. Be aware that your weight can fluctuate as much as 3-5 pounds every day. Food and water, plus bladder and bowel movements, as well as, perspiration and your cycle will make an enormous difference in your weight every day. Also, be sure to watch your salt intake and make sure you are drinking enough water every day.

Also, if no one has ever told you, there truly is only one correct way to weigh yourself. Given that you are going to be on a scale a lot, first, buy a scale that only you will use. Most scales work on spring system. Over time, the springs will wear out and give you a false reading and you will really be upset. A digital or analog scale might be the best scale for you.

Next, create a plan for daily weighing. Weigh yourself when your body is at its lowest weight for the day, and stick with that time. It should have been hours since you last ate. The morning works best for this.

So the morning that you start, wake up, use the bathroom and weigh yourself. Do it right away. You cannot have any food or other fluid in your system.

Stand square and straight-backed on your scale with even weight distribution in both of your feet. Breathe out to help yourself relax. Do not get dressed first; clothes add up to five to ten pounds of extra weight.

Motivate yourself to weigh yourself daily with a method that work for you. You can write a note to yourself and tape it near your bathroom mirror, then, leave the scale in a place where it can't be missed or set up a daily alarm on your cell phone as a reminder.

Remember that understanding how your weight fluctuates in response to food, mood and exercise on a daily basis will give you essential knowledge about your body, when you review the results. It will also give you an understanding of what works and what doesn't work, but then, prepare to be disturbed.

Sometimes, you will have to face the harsh realities of what you eat and how you eat in order to change the way that you eat. Don't be afraid to change the small things. The little changes can provide big results in your weight loss. This weight loss solution is not about me, it is about you. It's your life, it's your body and it's your health. It's time to take control of it.

You already know that this isn't easy. But, it is doable. You can do it. I did it. You can too. This journey to lose weight has the ability to make you either better or bitter. It can make you or break you. You can be the victim of your weight or the victor in healthy eating. I want you to win! This will make the next step quite simple. Now, let's begin to use what you have learned....

Sample of Your Daily Tracking System

	Date	Weigh In	Loss (-)/ Gain (+)
Day 4	6/8/12	165 Lbs.	-2 Lbs.

My goal is to weigh 150 pounds! I can do it!

Breakfast: a bagel with peanut butter and a glass of non-fat milk

Mid-morning snack: A granola bar and yogurt

Lunch: a turkey sandwich on honey wheat bread with lettuce and tomatoes, lite mayo and water

Mid-Day Snack: A handful of almonds and low-fat milk

Dinner: A rib eye steak, mashed potatoes and spinach, a glass of water

Exercise: I walked up the five flights to my office and parked at the other end of the lot.

Moods/Thoughts/Feelings:

I'm stressed. I have a big project coming up at work. Tomorrow, I am going to ask Sarah in accounting to walk with me after work.

Before You Begin Your First Seven Days, Say This Aloud Right Now, And, Then, Every Day Until You Know It By Heart And Believe In It:

I want to look better.

I want to eat better.

I want to feel better.

I want to have more energy.

I am losing this weight!

I can do this!

Your 7 Day Daily Tracking System

Day 1:	Date	Weigh In	Loss (-)/ Gain (+)
	_____	_____	_____

My goal is to weigh _____ pounds! I can do it.

Breakfast:

Mid-morning snack:

Lunch:

Mid-Day Snack:

Dinner:

Exercise:

Moods/Thoughts/Feelings:

Visualize Your Success...

Start visualizing how you will look when you reach your ideal or goal weight.

How will you feel when you lose the weight?

What will people say about you?

What will you say about your weight loss?

What will you be able to do more of?

Spend a few minutes thinking about this.

You will not be a victim of your weight.

Say it...I will be slimmer. Then, see your success!

Your 7 Day Daily Tracking System

	Date	Weigh In	Loss (-)/ Gain (+)
Day 2:			
	_____	_____	_____

My goal is to weigh _____ pounds! I can do it.

Breakfast:

Mid-morning snack:

Lunch:

Mid-Day Snack:

Dinner:

Exercise:

Moods/Thoughts/Feelings:

Stop Making Excuses!

Did you exercise at all today?

Did you skip or skimp on any meals?

Are you ready to lose weight?

Remember, if we are not honest with ourselves, how can we be real about losing weight?

Remember to take responsibility for your own choices and actions.

You are in control of your eating.

You are in control of your weight.

It's your life, your health and your body! No excuses!

Your 7 Day Daily Tracking System

		Loss (-)/
Day 3:	**Date** **Weigh In**	**Gain (+)**
	_____ _____	_____

My goal is to weigh _____ pounds! I can do it.

Breakfast:

Mid-morning snack:

Lunch:

Mid-Day Snack:

Dinner:

Exercise:

Moods/Thoughts/Feelings:

Lose Weight For You!

Nobody should care about your health more than you should care about it yourself.

Listen to your body's true hunger signs.

Your family and friends might be afraid that you will change too much from the person they know and already love.

Gradually lose the weight to introduce them to who you are supposed to be.

You may not always get the encouragement that you need or want from other people.

Losing weight allows you to live a longer, healthier and more fulfilling life.

You matter. You owe it to yourself to be healthier.

Your 7 Day Daily Tracking System

			Loss (-)/
Day 4:	Date	Weigh In	Gain (+)
	_____	_____	_____

My goal is to weigh _____ pounds! I can do it.

Breakfast:

Mid-morning snack:

Lunch:

Mid-Day Snack:

Dinner:

Exercise:

Moods/Thoughts/Feelings:

Losing Weight Shouldn't Be Kept Secret At All!

You should never be embarrassed about your decision to lose weight and eat healthier.

Be proud of yourself and your accomplishments.

When you are with your friends and family, tell them about your plans and ask for their help.

Stay focused, even when others try to stop you.

Don't be ashamed of your mistakes.

Your success is rooted in your failures; it will show you what not to do when you are trying to lose weight.

Tell the world! Or your body will tell them for you!

Your 7 Day Daily Tracking System

	Date	Weigh In	Loss (-)/ Gain (+)
Day 5:	_____	_____	_____

My goal is to weigh _____ **pounds! I can do it.**

Breakfast:

Mid-morning snack:

Lunch:

Mid-Day Snack:

Dinner:

Exercise:

Moods/Thoughts/Feelings:

Challenge Yourself!

Look at reaching your ideal weight as a challenge for yourself to see what you can really do when you are pushed to do it.

Look at this as an opportunity to learn something new about yourself and what you are capable of when challenged.

Push yourself to your uppermost limits.

You will never know what you can do, if you don't at least try to do something about it.

This will only make you stronger.

Each step in your exercising will build your self-confidence, motivation and your will power.

Never say the word "can't."

What you say that you can't do is what you won't do.

You can do it!

Your 7 Day Daily Tracking System

	Date	Weigh In	Loss (-)/ Gain (+)
Day 6:	_____	_____	_____

My goal is to weigh _____ pounds! I can do it.

Breakfast:

Mid-morning snack:

Lunch:

Mid-Day Snack:

Dinner:

Exercise:

Moods/Thoughts/Feelings:

Keep Going! Don't Stop!

Think about how far you have come.

Keep your goal to lose weight in mind.

If you miss a day of exercise, do it tomorrow.

This is helping to improve your life.

Feel the weight coming off.

You can't turn back now.

Remember your ideal goal weight.

Don't Give Up Now! Keep Going! Don't Stop Now!

Your 7 Day Daily Tracking System

			Loss (-)/
Day 7:	**Date**	**Weigh In**	**Gain (+)**
	_____	_____	_____

My goal is to weigh _____ pounds! I can do it.

Breakfast:

Mid-morning snack:

Lunch:

Mid-Day Snack:

Dinner:

Exercise:

Moods/Thoughts/Feelings:

Right Now, How Do You Feel?

The first seven days tend to be rough. Being overweight, your body has had to work harder to support that extra weight. So how did you do? If you have lost even a half of a pound to two pounds in this first seven days, you are off to a good start. Keep going! If you have or haven't, then here is the point where we need to talk.

From time to time, you might have to refer to this part of the book, regardless if you are losing the weight or not. This will help you stay focused. Remember that nobody is expecting you to be perfect in trying to lose weight. When you mess up, or haven't lost as much weight as you thought you should have, and we all have, or will, at some point feel like this...learn from it.

So what you ate that Double fudge brownie that your sister made. It is just a setback, not the end of the world. Give yourself room to breathe. You should never berate yourself for anything involving your weight. When you make a mistake, own up to it and move on. When you are walking around feeling better and looking better, you won't worry about that brownie then.

Also, when that happens I need you to do something more important. I need you to practice the greatest thing that nobody has ever bothered to put into a diet—forgiveness. Nobody is perfect. That's why you should forgive yourself and forgive what you did. Forgive yourself even for all of the years that you struggled with your weight. You now know better and can do better.

Everyone makes a mistake, that's why any teacher will tell you that God made erasers. Never be too hard on yourself. Always, celebrate your success. Don't dwell on your failures. They aren't real failures; they are lessons that will remind you that you just have to do better.

Even if you put back on those five pounds that you worked so hard to lose, say to yourself, "I lost those five pounds and I can do it again." The key to any successful weight loss is awareness. Awareness brings about change. When you know better, you can do better. If you want to lose weight, just make better choices.

In keeping track, you will also begin to notice if you gained any weight because of the foods that you were eating. If you lost any weight, you will keep what you have been doing going. You will also begin to see the feelings that were associated with the days you gained weight and will try to avoid them.

The one thing that I didn't do, if you didn't notice it, was tell you the exact times when you should eat. You have to decide that. You have been trained since childhood to eat at certain points in their day. In the morning, you should eat breakfast. At noon, you should eat lunch. Then, around six, you should eat dinner. Start eating when you are hungry. Stop eating when you are feeling full. Don't think about it. Just stop.

Now that you have learned how to eat for a week, let's do it for another 30 days, and then, for good. If doing anything 21 times makes a habit, I wanted to make sure this one lasts. Be sure to share your successes with me via my website www.HungryChickDiet.com. I wish you the best of luck to you in everything that you do...

175

Don't Forget To Say This Aloud Every Day Until You Know It By Heart And Believe In It:

I want to look better.

I want to eat better.

I want to feel better.

I want to have more energy.

I AM losing this weight!

I can do this!

Your 30 Day Daily Tracking System

			Loss (-)/
Day 1:	**Date**	**Weigh In**	**Gain (+)**
	_____	_____	_____

My goal is to weigh _____ pounds! I can do it!

Breakfast:

Mid-morning snack:

Lunch:

Mid-Day Snack:

Dinner:

Exercise:

Moods/Thoughts/Feelings:

Your 30 Day Daily Tracking System

	Date	Weigh In	Loss (-)/ Gain (+)
Day 2:	_____	_____	_____

My goal is to weigh _____ pounds! I can do it!

Breakfast:

Mid-morning snack:

Lunch:

Mid-Day Snack:

Dinner:

Exercise:

Moods/Thoughts/Feelings:

Your 30 Day Daily Tracking System

	Date	Weigh In	Loss (-)/ Gain (+)
Day 3:	_____	_____	_____

My goal is to weigh _____ pounds! I can do it!

Breakfast:

Mid-morning snack:

Lunch:

Mid-Day Snack:

Dinner:

Exercise:

Moods/Thoughts/Feelings:

Your 30 Day Daily Tracking System

Day 4:	Date	Weigh In	Loss (-)/ Gain (+)
	_____	_____	_____

My goal is to weigh _____ pounds! I can do it!

Breakfast:

Mid-morning snack:

Lunch:

Mid-Day Snack:

Dinner:

Exercise:

Moods/Thoughts/Feelings:

Your 30 Day Daily Tracking System

			Loss (-)/
Day 5:	**Date**	**Weigh In**	**Gain (+)**
	_____	_____	_____

My goal is to weigh _____ pounds! I can do it!

Breakfast:

Mid-morning snack:

Lunch:

Mid-Day Snack:

Dinner:

Exercise:

Moods/Thoughts/Feelings:

Your 30 Day Daily Tracking System

	Date	Weigh In	Loss (-)/ Gain (+)
Day 6:			
	_____	_____	_____

My goal is to weigh _____ pounds! I can do it!

Breakfast:

Mid-morning snack:

Lunch:

Mid-Day Snack:

Dinner:

Exercise:

Moods/Thoughts/Feelings:

Your 30 Day Daily Tracking System

	Loss (-)/

Day 7:   **Date**   **Weigh In**   **Loss (-)/ Gain (+)**

_____   _____   _____

My goal is to weigh _____ pounds! I can do it!

Breakfast:

Mid-morning snack:

Lunch:

Mid-Day Snack:

Dinner:

Exercise:

Moods/Thoughts/Feelings:

Your 30 Day Daily Tracking System

Day 8:	Date	Weigh In	Loss (-)/ Gain (+)
	_____	_____	_____

My goal is to weigh _____ pounds! I can do it!

Breakfast:

Mid-morning snack:

Lunch:

Mid-Day Snack:

Dinner:

Exercise:

Moods/Thoughts/Feelings:

Your 30 Day Daily Tracking System

	Date	Weigh In	Loss (-)/ Gain (+)
Day 9:	____	_____	_____

My goal is to weigh _____ pounds! I can do it!

Breakfast:

Mid-morning snack:

Lunch:

Mid-Day Snack:

Dinner:

Exercise:

Moods/Thoughts/Feelings:

Your 30 Day Daily Tracking System

Day 10:	Date	Weigh In	Loss (-)/ Gain (+)
	_____	_____	_____

My goal is to weigh _____ pounds! I can do it!

Breakfast:

Mid-morning snack:

Lunch:

Mid-Day Snack:

Dinner:

Exercise:

Moods/Thoughts/Feelings:

Your 30 Day Daily Tracking System

			Loss (-)/
Day 11:	**Date**	**Weigh In**	**Gain (+)**
	_____	_____	_____

My goal is to weigh _____ pounds! I can do it!

Breakfast:

Mid-morning snack:

Lunch:

Mid-Day Snack:

Dinner:

Exercise:

Moods/Thoughts/Feelings:

Your 30 Day Daily Tracking System

		Loss (-)/
Day 12:	**Date**	**Weigh In**	**Gain (+)**
	_____	_____	_____

My goal is to weigh _____ pounds! I can do it!

Breakfast:

Mid-morning snack:

Lunch:

Mid-Day Snack:

Dinner:

Exercise:

Moods/Thoughts/Feelings:

Your 30 Day Daily Tracking System

	Date	Weigh In	Loss (-)/ Gain (+)
Day 13:	_____	_____	_____

My goal is to weigh _____ pounds! I can do it!

Breakfast:

Mid-morning snack:

Lunch:

Mid-Day Snack:

Dinner:

Exercise:

Moods/Thoughts/Feelings:

Your 30 Day Daily Tracking System

	Date	Weigh In	Loss (-)/ Gain (+)
Day 14:	_____	_____	_____

My goal is to weigh _____ pounds! I can do it!

Breakfast:

Mid-morning snack:

Lunch:

Mid-Day Snack:

Dinner:

Exercise:

Moods/Thoughts/Feelings:

Your 30 Day Daily Tracking System

			Loss (-)/
Day 15:	**Date**	**Weigh In**	**Gain (+)**
	_____	_____	_____

My goal is to weigh _____ pounds! I can do it!

Breakfast:

Mid-morning snack:

Lunch:

Mid-Day Snack:

Dinner:

Exercise:

Moods/Thoughts/Feelings:

Your 30 Day Daily Tracking System

		Loss (-)/
Day 16:	**Date** **Weigh In**	**Gain (+)**
	_____ _____	_____

My goal is to weigh _____ **pounds! I can do it!**

Breakfast:

Mid-morning snack:

Lunch:

207

Mid-Day Snack:

Dinner:

Exercise:

Moods/Thoughts/Feelings:

Your 30 Day Daily Tracking System

	Date	Weigh In	Loss (-)/ Gain (+)
Day 17:	_____	_____	_____

My goal is to weigh _____ pounds! I can do it!

Breakfast:

Mid-morning snack:

Lunch:

Mid-Day Snack:

Dinner:

Exercise:

Moods/Thoughts/Feelings:

Your 30 Day Daily Tracking System

		Loss (-)/
Day 18:	Date	Weigh In	Gain (+)

_____   _____   _____

My goal is to weigh _____ **pounds! I can do it!**

Breakfast:

Mid-morning snack:

Lunch:

Mid-Day Snack:

Dinner:

Exercise:

Moods/Thoughts/Feelings:

Your 30 Day Daily Tracking System

			Loss (-)/
Day 19:	**Date**	**Weigh In**	**Gain (+)**
	_____	_____	_____

My goal is to weigh _____ pounds! I can do it!

Breakfast:

Mid-morning snack:

Lunch:

Mid-Day Snack:

Dinner:

Exercise:

Moods/Thoughts/Feelings:

Your 30 Day Daily Tracking System

	Date	Weigh In	Loss (-)/ Gain (+)
Day 20:	_____	_____	_____

My goal is to weigh _____ pounds! I can do it!

Breakfast:

Mid-morning snack:

Lunch:

Mid-Day Snack:

Dinner:

Exercise:

Moods/Thoughts/Feelings:

Your 30 Day Daily Tracking System

			Loss (-)/
Day 21:	Date	Weigh In	Gain (+)
	_____	_____	_____

My goal is to weigh _____ pounds! I can do it!

Breakfast:

Mid-morning snack:

Lunch:

Mid-Day Snack:

Dinner:

Exercise:

Moods/Thoughts/Feelings:

Your 30 Day Daily Tracking System

Day 22:	Date	Weigh In	Loss (-)/ Gain (+)
	_____	_____	_____

My goal is to weigh _____ pounds! I can do it!

Breakfast:

Mid-morning snack:

Lunch:

Mid-Day Snack:

Dinner:

Exercise:

Moods/Thoughts/Feelings:

Your 30 Day Daily Tracking System

		Loss (-)/
Day 23:	**Date**	**Weigh In**	**Gain (+)**

_____ _____ _____

My goal is to weigh _____ pounds! I can do it!

Breakfast:

Mid-morning snack:

Lunch:

Mid-Day Snack:

Dinner:

Exercise:

Moods/Thoughts/Feelings:

Your 30 Day Daily Tracking System

			Loss (-)/
Day 24:	Date	Weigh In	Gain (+)
	_____	_____	_____

My goal is to weigh _____ pounds! I can do it!

Breakfast:

Mid-morning snack:

Lunch:

Mid-Day Snack:

Dinner:

Exercise:

Moods/Thoughts/Feelings:

Your 30 Day Daily Tracking System

	Loss (-)/		
Day 25:	Date	Weigh In	Gain (+)
	_____	_____	_____

My goal is to weigh _____ pounds! I can do it!

Breakfast:

Mid-morning snack:

Lunch:

Mid-Day Snack:

Dinner:

Exercise:

Moods/Thoughts/Feelings:

Your 30 Day Daily Tracking System

		Loss (-)/
Day 26:	**Date** **Weigh In**	**Gain (+)**

_____	_____	_____

My goal is to weigh _____ **pounds! I can do it!**

Breakfast:

Mid-morning snack:

Lunch:

Mid-Day Snack:

Dinner:

Exercise:

Moods/Thoughts/Feelings:

Your 30 Day Daily Tracking System

			Loss (-)/
Day 27:	Date	Weigh In	Gain (+)
	_____	_____	_____

My goal is to weigh _____ pounds! I can do it!

Breakfast:

Mid-morning snack:

Lunch:

Mid-Day Snack:

Dinner:

Exercise:

Moods/Thoughts/Feelings:

Your 30 Day Daily Tracking System

		Loss (-)/
Day 28:	**Date** **Weigh In**	**Gain (+)**
	_____ _____	_____

My goal is to weigh _____ **pounds! I can do it!**

Breakfast:

Mid-morning snack:

Lunch:

Mid-Day Snack:

Dinner:

Exercise:

Moods/Thoughts/Feelings:

Your 30 Day Daily Tracking System

Day 29:	Date	Weigh In	Loss (-)/ Gain (+)
	_____	_____	_____

My goal is to weigh _____ pounds! I can do it!

Breakfast:

Mid-morning snack:

Lunch:

Mid-Day Snack:

Dinner:

Exercise:

Moods/Thoughts/Feelings:

Your 30 Day Daily Tracking System

			Loss (-)/
Day 30:	**Date**	**Weigh In**	**Gain (+)**
	_____	_____	_____

My goal is to weigh _____ pounds! I can do it!

Breakfast:

Mid-morning snack:

Lunch:

Mid-Day Snack:

Dinner:

Exercise:

Moods/Thoughts/Feelings:

Congratulate Yourself!

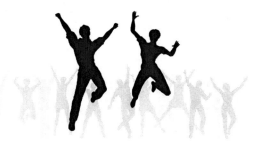

If you can do this for just 30 days, you can do this for the rest of your life. Remember to…

- ✓ Make healthier choices in your meals
- ✓ Eat early and eat often
- ✓ Eat when hungry, stop when full
- ✓ Drink enough water every single day
- ✓ Watch your portion sizes at all times
- ✓ Add spice to your food, not salt
- ✓ Use non-food stress relievers
- ✓ Keep active to keep physically fit
- ✓ When you need it, seek help or support
- ✓ Always follow your doctor's advice

Keep this book on your bedside as a friendly reminder of what you have accomplished.

You Did It! Keep Going!

About Chef Jai Scovers…

Chef Jai Scovers (pronounced Jay Scoh-Vers) is a trained gourmet chef and a graduate of the world famous Restaurant School at Walnut Hill College in Philadelphia, Pennsylvania, where she was trained in every aspect of the food industry, including food selection, recipe development and menu planning and the nutritional value of food.

Chef Jai has worked to develop her skills in such well-known and recognized dining establishments, as the famed Stephen Starr restaurants to Harrah's Showboat Hotel and Casino in Atlantic City, New Jersey.

She currently holds her nationally recognized ServSafe certification. This certification demonstrates her ability and commitment to food safety, in the areas of food storage, preparation, cleaning, sanitizing and cooking.

Chef Jai Scovers is an advocate in the fight against preventing food borne illnesses and raising awareness about healthy eating. Awareness brings about change. She is also a supporter of several women based charities and fighting childhood hunger.

Proceeds from the sale of every copy of this book sold will go to support several charitable efforts, including, but not limited to, the race to find a cure for breast cancer, ending domestic violence and supporting local food banks to feed hungry families. Thank you for your support. Your support will allow these charities to help so many more people.

Index

CPSIA information can be obtained
at www.ICGtesting.com
Printed in the USA
FSOW02n1050110117
29519FS

9 780979 930232